STAGESTRUCK

Kristin Kopstich
Photo 1998

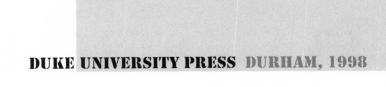

DUKE UNIVERSITY PRESS DURHAM, 1998

SARAH SCHULMAN

Theater,

AIDS, and

the

Marketing

of

Gay America

STAGESTRUCK

© 1998 Sarah Schulman, Inc.

This edition © 1998 Duke University Press

All rights reserved

Printed in the United States of America on acid-free

paper ⊚

Typeset in Times Roman with Stencil display

by Tseng Information Systems, Inc.

Library of Congress Cataloging-in-Publication Data

appear on the last printed page of this book.

Also by Sarah Schulman

For

carlos ricardo martinez

and

Jeff Weiss

My shame was only exceeded by my fury.

—Bette Davis

Broadway

NOVEL APPROACH TO A DOWNTOWN MUSICAL *

by Dudley Saunders

Puccini may not be around to demand his share of the credit for *Rent,* but plenty of folks among the living are. These days, people are talking about some remarkable similarities between the hit musical and Sarah Schulman's novel *People In Trouble.*

Published shortly after Jonathan Larson and Billy Aronson began working on the rock opera, *People In Trouble* was (and remains) the only novel about East Village artists grappling with AIDS and homelessness. According to Aronson, who parted company with Larson early on, only one of the plotlines in *Rent*—its central *La Boheme*-inspired love story—was in place when he and Larson collaborated. Later, however, Larson's script picked up some interesting parallels with *People In Trouble.*

In the novel, Kate, a selfish East Village artist at the end of a relationship with a male artist, falls in love with a lesbian social activist. Kate's performance-art piece leads to a riot that brings down a greedy landlord trying to evict people with AIDS.

In *Rent,* Maureen, a selfish East Village artist at the end of a relationship with a male artist, falls in love with a lesbian social activist. Later, Maureen's performance piece targeting a greedy landlord trying to evict people with AIDS leads to a riot.

People In Trouble features an interracial gay couple named James and Scott, one an AIDS activist, the other a drag queen, both HIV-positive, one of whom dies. Ditto, *Rent,* where they are named Tom and Angel. At one point in the novel, James and Scott use stolen credit card numbers to charge groceries for the poor; in the musical, Tom rewires a grocery store cash machine to give food money to the poor.

Schulman is angrier about the depiction in *Rent* of gay people and the AIDS crisis than any allegedly lifted material.

"The message of my novel is that personal homophobia becomes societal neglect, that there is a direct relationship between the two," she insists. "The message of *Rent* is quite the opposite, that straight people are the heroic center of the AIDS crisis."

That interpretation, however, may owe more to the contribution of dramaturg Lynn Thompson than to Larson. She is suing for a share of *Rent*'s sizable profits: reading through her lawsuit one is struck by just how much of the "message" she takes credit for: focusing on the heterosexual love story, reducing the number of H I V-positive characters, purging the show of "unsympathetic" emotions to make it "positive, life affirming."

Indeed, Thomson's description of Larson's original suggests a far more accurate portrait of A I D S-afflicted artists—one that probably wouldn't have appealed to Broadway audiences.

Larson arranged to share credit and part of the *Rent* windfall with Aronson and, Thompson claims, planned to do the same for her. And perhaps he had something similar in. mind for Schulman: Larson announced his debt to *People In Trouble* to at least one prominent theater professional back in 1994, someone who has promised to come forward in the event of another lawsuit.

CONTENTS

ACKNOWLEDGMENTS

Various parts of this work appeared in earlier versions in
*The Progressive, Lambda Book Report, Harvard Gay and Lesbian Review,
Gay Community News,* and *New York Press,* and in the form of lectures.
Thanks to Don Shewey, Maxine Wolfe, Michael Bronski, Dudley Saunders,
Chris Straayer, Larry Gross, the Millay Colony, and the MacDowell Colony.
Deep appreciation to William Clark for engaging this material on the level
of art and ideas. Special thanks to Carrie Moyer for her expertise and
organic understanding of the issues at hand. Gratitude to my editor
Richard Morrison at Duke University Press for his thorough
reading, thoughtful suggestions, and insights.

INTRODUCTION

My mother says that I am always looking for trouble. But even she had to admit that this time trouble came looking for me. From the first moment I realized that the Broadway musical *Rent* contained characters, events, and paradigms from my 1990 novel, *People in Trouble,* I knew I was in the middle of a mess. But I had no idea of how messy this mess would become. For it was revealed as much more than a simple case of plagiarism.

As the months, and then years, unfolded, I experienced this event in many different ways. At first I just wanted to protect my copyright. It all seemed quite clear. My material had been published; it appeared in *Rent.* My novel was about the impact of personal homophobia on the broader AIDS crisis. *Rent* was about how straight people were the heroes of AIDS. All I had to do was go to court and I would get credit and money and bring to the surface a crucial discussion about how AIDS was going to be represented in this society.

But as I gathered more and more evidence about the protective institutions encircling *Rent* and about the ways my work had been lifted, it became clear that legal justice would elude me. I simply was not powerful enough. At that point of revelation, there was a profound shift in my thinking. Even though, at times, legal action seemed impossible and therefore the fantasy of money and credit disappeared, I realized that the outstanding moral and historical questions at the center of this case corresponded with those at the core of my own personal journey.

One of the many things I've learned from this experience is how the miraculous movement of history can converge on one moment in an individual's life. I saw that this coincidence—the collision of my personal work with a social trend of artifice—was an exceptional opportunity through which to understand recent historical shifts. This was particularly engaging for me, because the props were the commodification of ideas about AIDS, homosexuality, neighborhood, artistic production, and theater—the very themes that had long been at the center of my life. The questions I found myself asking were stark ones. How is AIDS going to be represented in this society? What is the result of the cultural appropriation of gay and lesbian work? What happens when an individual artist is dominated by a corporate product? What is the impact of the current culture of art-making on these questions?

In Part One, "The Dirt," I will tell the gossip: who said what to whom, who did what to whom, the amazing amount of subterfuge that one billion dollars in assets can produce. I will try to piece together the sequence of events concerning the unauthorized use of my materials in the production of *Rent* and what happened when I tried to do something about it. Here are the acts of kindness and integrity, side by side with the dismissals and humiliations I found along the way; what happened when I tried to take on hugely powerful people; and what I learned in the process.

In this book I will try to address these subjects within a number of frameworks. In Part Two, "Simulacra, Authenticity, and the Theatrical Context of *Rent*," I will look at the 1995–96 theatrical season in New York City, the setting for the opening of *Rent* at New York Theater Workshop and its subsequent move to Broadway. I will examine what other plays opened that season, especially plays written by the very people *Rent* claims to represent. What were Black women saying about themselves? What were gay men with HIV saying about themselves? What was the context of representation of homosexuality, race, and marginality on the New York stage? Here

I hope to contrast how the people profitably described in *Rent* actually represented themselves at the same theatrical moment that *Rent* came on the scene. And I will underline the implications of the dramatic differences.

Part Three, "Selling A I D S and Other Consequences of the Commodification of Homosexuality," tries to untangle how a country devastated by the A I D S crisis can embrace a play that sinisterly distorts the history of A I D S. Here I analyze the emergence of gay people as a consumer group to be niche-marketed to and the rise of gay images in advertising aimed at the general market. I want to understand the relationship between these palatable, untrue images and the ability of the country to embrace equally untrue stories about the A I D S crisis. This process gives me the opportunity to go further and try to untangle the relationship between advertising and contemporary debates about homosexuality, such as the value of a gay nuclear family ideal or the rise of biological determinist theories. I am particularly interested in the marketing opportunities these social developments provide.

Finally, in the conclusion, "The Creation of a Fake, Public Homosexuality," I look at the function of gay images produced by and for straight people and the strange impact of these images on gay audiences. At the core of my thinking is the belief that the presumably "objective" stance of the dominant culture is artificial and not, in fact, objective. Challenging their *feelings* of neutrality is essential for any truthful expression to emerge.

For me, the fundamental difference between corporate product and art is that art is an engagement with the parts of a human being that are unique, difficult to express, and essential to understand. My own process as a novelist for the last fifteen years involves facing a difficult idea or emotion that many people do not want to face, and going so far with it as to provoke an emotional catharsis that results in a revelation. When the writing is completed, the author offers this revelation as a gift to the reader. Corporate product is the opposite of art, because it denies the value of eccentric investigation. In other words, I offer you this book and hope that it gives you something worth thinking about, because, even if it doesn't produce money, it can produce a level of inquiry that is really interesting. And that would make this whole process ultimately worthwhile.

RENT: THE DIRT

PART 1

Here's what happened: I was twenty-eight years old in 1987, the year I joined ACT UP (the just-born AIDS Coalition To Unleash Power) and full throttle into a love affair with a married woman. An artist, she was very conflicted about her sexuality with women and had contempt for the gay community in general. She practiced an art ideology that equated formal invention with radical content, something I contested passionately. My fantasy was that by exposing her to the realities of the AIDS crisis, she would drop her blinders about the functions of homophobia and simultaneously develop an understanding of the value of artwork rooted in experience. Needless to say, older now, I understand that my project was doomed from the start.

That year I completed my fourth novel, *People in Trouble,* about a triangle composed of a married artist couple and the woman's younger lesbian lover. The novel was set against the backdrop of the AIDS crisis and featured many scenes and feelings that came directly out of my actual experience. *People in Trouble* is about an East Village performance artist who is at the end of a relationship with a male artist and who, despite her own homophobia, falls in love with a lesbian. She creates a performance piece that targets a greedy landlord who is evicting people with AIDS. There is a subplot about an interracial gay male couple—one a queen, one an activist—in which one dies of AIDS. A second subplot involves an AIDS-activist group called Justice, who devise a credit card scam to feed homeless people. It was, as David Leavitt wrote in 1990, "the first work of fiction that portrays the enormous activist response the epidemic has generated." And the book clearly showed how this response was rooted in the gay and lesbian community, despite the neglect and inaction of dominant society.

While I was writing the novel, I met Stewart Wallace, a composer who was finishing his score for an operatic collaboration called *Where's Dick?* with librettist Michael Korie, to be directed by Richard Foreman.

Stewart and I talked a lot about A I D S, and a short time later he and Michael offered to collaborate on an operatic adaptation of *People in Trouble* for a prominent American opera house, also to be directed by Foreman. It would be the first A I D S opera for a closeted but A I D S-devastated opera world. We worked for a while on a treatment for the piece and came up with one that opened with a romantic duet for two female voices. But when they presented the treatment to the director of the opera, he panicked.

"I can't have dripping pussies on my stage," he said. "These women are not heroic."

And so our project was dropped, and Stewart and Michael went on to write the acclaimed opera *Harvey Milk,* featuring a male hero, which was subsequently recorded and played successfully in New York (at the New York City Opera), San Francisco, and Europe.

Michael, however, was still interested in pursuing *People in Trouble,* and he sent copies of the manuscript, the galleys, and finally, in 1990, the published book to a variety of composers, directors, and producers in New York and Europe. At that time there was no context for work with primary lesbian content at the level of production that we sought, and homophobia was still either ignored or soft-pedaled in the theater and on film. Although the treatment and novel went to a number of highly respected producers including Joanne Akalaitis at the Public Theater, Joe Melillo at the Brooklyn Academy of Music, and Ira Weitzman at Lincoln Center among others, the response was less than enthusiastic. The Public lost our materials three times, and even though they were replaced three times, they actually never officially responded. Most other venues simply said no. But some of the reactions were as shocking and prejudiced as that of the misogynist opera queen of the story. For example there was the famous gay male composer who turned us down because he said he couldn't write romantic music for two women. Then there was the straight woman director who was not sympathetic to the AIDS content. "Straight people have problems too, you know," she said. "My niece and her husband can't find a large enough apartment." Michael was still enthusiastic about the script and felt that it could be "a *West Side Story* for the 90s," "a modern *La Bohème*," both phrases that we used in our pitch. At one point David Van Tieghem, the composer, agreed to work on the piece. But, by 1992 we had given up: the social environment was too conservative for a heroic opera about AIDS with a lesbian protagonist. It probably still is. That year, the book was optioned for film by two openly lesbian television writers, but they, too, underestimated the level of prejudice, and despite being very well connected, they could not find investors interested in bringing a story of the AIDS crisis from a lesbian perspective to the screen. The book stayed in print but, aside from three foreign editions, received no further attention.

In February 1996, Don Shewey and I were writing a column together for the *New York Press* (see Part Two). We went to review the new musical *Rent,* which had opened the previous night at New York Theater Workshop. The author-composer Jonathan Larson had died before the first preview, and a huge amount of tension, sadness, hype, and expectation was placed on what might otherwise have been a small run at a downtown theater.

It was seven years since my novel had been published. I hadn't read it since going through the final galleys. I had written three novels, four plays, and one nonfiction book since that time, and the characters and details of *People in Trouble* were far out of my mind.

Yet, when I sat in the audience at *Rent,* I felt a creeping resentment. I remember sitting there thinking, *Now they're stealing from us.* I identified with, or recognized something about, the play even though I despised it. And I remember berating myself for feeling jealous or ripped off, resolving to keep those feelings under wraps when I wrote the review. I worried that my emotional reaction was inappropriate because I didn't understand where it was coming from.

Don Shewey and I wrote the only two bad reviews that *Rent* got in all of New York. Just for the record, I will reproduce mine here.

RENT BY SARAH SCHULMAN — February 22, 1996

These kids grew up wanting to be Irene Cara singing "I'm gonna live forever." They are the teenage Puerto Rican drag queens and home girls who wanted to be pop stars, movie stars, to sing in large airy theaters to adoring crowds. You can see them do that at New York Theater Workshop and then, when the show moves, on Broadway. The cast of *Rent* is the most intoxicating and vulnerable element of the show. Otherwise this musical about life in the East Village, based on the plot of *La Boheme,* is a bit flat.

It's hard to know how to really look at this piece. The music telegraphs *energy, energy, youth, vigor,* but after a while some of the score sounds like it could be an ad for Diet Coke. Is that a problem? Do we expect musical scores to be more than upbeat generic pop? If the standard is comfortable entertainment, that explains why *Rent* is such a big hit. If you want more from theater you may be disappointed.

As a writer who's lived in and recorded the East Village for 12 years, I immediately recognized and appreciated particular moments from the culture. Those tables in cheap restaurants with 20 friends and 13 orders of french fries, filled with love and exuberance after somebody's show. The battle of privilege and ego between a lesbian and her lover's ex-boyfriend is one of those daily East Village occurrences that I've never seen represented on stage before. Finding your own stuff for sale on St. Marks Pl. These moments gave me that pang of joyful recognition that comes from witnessing my own experiences onstage, something I almost never see. All those plays Don and I go to always seem to be about somebody else.

But always gnawing at my mind during this play was the now-daily experience of watching gay artists slightly shift or reposition their subjectivity to achieve broader professional success. I am obsessed by this. It is my version of the Kennedy assassination. It is a conspiracy.

The central relationship in *Rent* is between two men, "roommates," both "straight," but Roger (Adam Pascal) has A I D S, immediately explained by the fact that he used to be a junkie. Obviously the emotional motive for this play was a relationship between two white men who share their lives together. Why do they have to be straight?

The main subplot is Roger falling in love with Mimi, an active junkie, but their love conquers all. The gay people get the sub-subplots: a black man and a Puerto Rican drag queen fall in love, and the queen dies. Mark, the HIV-negative guy, lost his white girlfriend Maureen when she fell in love with Joanne, a black lesbian, but all they do is fight. They never seem to help each other or heal or transform each other. The love stories get pretty banal and are only sparked by energetic performances from the gorgeous Fredi Walker as Joanne, sexy and warm-throated Adam Pascal and the sad, convincing Jesse L. Martin.

The shifting of centrality from gay to straight characters backfires, because Larson's heart is clearly with the queers. The most complex and moving sections of the play are those having to do with A I D S. The plot machinations about evictions, performance art and poverty are far less compelling. So the problem that the repositioning of gay characters inflicts on the larger piece is that its heart and soul are removed from the center. It becomes an esthetic problem, not an ideological one.

Once this whitewashing is set into place, a strange Benetton-like sheen comes over the plot. Suddenly Puerto Rican drag queens with A I D S, straight video artists from Scarsdale and black lesbians from upper-class families are all equal. They are all "La Vie Boheme." My experience of the various subcultures of East Village life is that they overlap on different occasions in various and complex ways, but they are not at all fully integrated. Very different kinds of people with very different kinds of access occupy parallel universes on the very same streets. When *Rent* loses its specificities, it loses its meaning. We know why artists and gay people are on the fringes of society, but what about all the others?

By placing a dominant culture hero at the center of his human landscape, Larson forces himself into focusing on a banal dilemma for Mark to resolve. In this case, M T V is calling and wants Mark to sell his video footage of an Ave. A riot. But he doesn't want to sell out. It amazes me that the two things theater seems unable to address are how political people function and how artists really live. If Larson's point is that for the fully privileged the phone call inevitably comes, while those with essential contributions to make to the culture are obstructed at every turn, this is not clear. Instead, he reinforces in the audience's mind that financial reward is a simple choice available to every nitwit with a camera.

In a sense *Rent* gives New Yorkers a comfortable image of themselves. People suffer because they have a romanticized self-image. They like it and they deserve it. C'est la vie. We're all the same anyway and we all really get along. Everything is really fine. Isn't it great to see such talented Latin actors on stage? A I D S is so sad, but straight love is real love, what a relief. Coke after Coke after Coke after Coke.

ACT ONE

You see, I thought that Jonathan Larson was gay and that he had died of A I D S. What else do white men die of at thirty-five in my universe? Actually, he was straight and died of an aortic aneurysm. But there was enough authenticity to some of the gay and A I D S details that I attributed it to him, not to me. Only later was I to understand that too many of those details came from my own book.

About a month later I was talking to Michael Korie on the phone.

"You must be so upset about *Rent,*" he said.

He then proceeded to tell me that in 1994 he had attended the Richard Rodgers Awards Dinner where he and Jonathan Larson were both being celebrated. Larson had told Michael that he was writing a musical about "bohemians on the Lower Eastside."

"Oh, have you read *People in Trouble,* by Sarah Schulman?" Michael asked.

"Yes," Larson said. "I'm using it."

Immediately, I went back and reread the novel. There was my plot, interwoven with *La Bohème.* Basically *Rent* had two plots: the straight half was from Puccini, and the gay half was from me. It was all there in Larson's version, but twisted. Whereas my story of the love triangle was told from the lesbian's point of view, Larson had turned the perspective so that the same triangle with the same plot points was being told from the straight man's point of view. While relying on my work for structure and content, he had transformed it into a dominant-culture piece by removing the lesbian authorial voice. Given how much obstruction I had faced in my fifteen years in print for having lesbian protagonists, this was a real slap in the face. It proved, what I had always known all along, that the characters, action, and dynamics of my novels were fine — only the lesbian protagonists kept me marginalized. Larson had moved the lesbian down to a secondary spot, and he had a hit with my ideas. Furthermore, it was a hit made possible only because of the groundwork set by actual gay and lesbian artists who had taken such pains to familiarize the heterosexual majority with our own existence. It was like a Mississippi bluesman having his song ripped off by Pat Boone. The very thing about it that made it commodifiable was the mediocrity that remained once the music's soul was stripped.

There was the scene between the lesbian and the husband in the book that had come directly from a real experience I'd had with my lover's husband on the street. No wonder I had praised the authenticity of the same encounter when it happened in the play! There was the same love triangle, there were the same subplots. There was the landlord, the political action. It was all there. In my book there was an interracial gay male couple, one an activist and a queen, the other HIV-positive and who dies of AIDS. In the play there was an interracial gay male couple; one was an activist, but the one who was HIV-positive and died of AIDS was the queen. It seemed like the unthinkable had happened. *Rent* was a direct rip-off of my book.

I started to try to find out some things about Jonathan Larson, whom I had never met or even heard of. I know a lot of things about him by now, most importantly that he was straight, that he'd only lived in the East Village for a few years. He was known for not being able to write plot or narrative structure. He'd had close friends with AIDS but was never in the ACT UP milieu. It just became more and more obvious that he had not had the lived experiences at the base of the play, and I had. Someone told me he had had a girl-friend who'd left him for a woman, which would have given him special interest in my novel. When I was writing *People in Trouble,* I'd always wondered if straight men (the handful that could bring themselves to read a novel with a lesbian protagonist) could iden-tify with the straight male character. This proved that they could, as long as the character was repositioned as the universal center.

My first step was to call the woman who had edited the novel at Dutton/Penguin. I left an extensive message with her assistant, but my editor never returned my call. After waiting too long I called the Penguin's legal department directly.

"I think someone has taken one of my properties," I told the woman on the other end of the phone. "Here's the plot of my novel. There's a love triangle against the backdrop of the AIDS crisis . . ."

"Are you talking about *Rent?*" she asked.

I wrote out a point-by-point comparison between the book and the play and faxed it to her, then faxed a copy to the editor, who still did not reply. I recapped the exact similarities between *People in Trouble* and *Rent.*

14

- Both are set in the East Village milieu of A I D S, homelessness, homosexuality, and artists.
- Both are about a love triangle between a straight artist couple and the woman's lesbian lover.
- The woman in the middle, in both pieces, is a performance artist who does a performance that defeats the greedy landlord evicting people with A I D S, which serves as a cathartic plot point for both works. In *People in Trouble* the landlord dies, in *Rent,* he changes his ways.
- In both pieces there is an interracial gay male couple where one partner dies of A I D S. In both works this death is a cathartic plot point.
- Both contain a scene where the lesbian meets the straight guy and they form some kind of strained relationship.
- In both, the lesbian couple become involved with people organizing to defend people with A I D S. In *People in Trouble* an A I D S activist group steals credit cards to feed the poor. In *Rent,* a gay man programs an A T M machine for similar purposes.

A few days later the woman from Legal called me back. She said that the similarities were startling but that when my literary agent, Diane Cleaver, had negotiated my contract, she had withheld theatrical rights because we were anticipating the *People in Trouble* opera. So the publisher had no contractual involvement in a case of theft of theatrical rights. I asked what would happen if they ever published *Rent* as a book or made a C D or movie out of it. She told me to talk to my agent.

That was all well and good, but Diane Cleaver, my literary agent for eight years, had died suddenly the previous April. So, I called the junior agent at her agency, who had inherited my file. This woman (I'll call her Morticia) had never met me, had never seen *Rent,* and had not read my book. Furthermore she had no interest in ever doing any of the above.

"There are a lot of novels about A I D S and the homeless and artists and gay people in the East Village," she said.

"Yeah," I said. "They're all by me."

"Forget about it," was her advice. Later she would write me a letter saying that she only wanted to work with writers who were "young, white males of British origin."

So, institutionally, I was screwed. I called a few people for advice about lawyers. A number of them referred me to lawyers who cost $220 an hour for a consultation. Since I had been buying groceries on credit cards for two years, that was out of the question.

I went to an activist lawyer who I had known from politics. She had also been a good friend of Diane's and had come up to me at the funeral and offered her services if I "ever needed anything." I told her the details of the case. She asked for a copy of the novel and said she would read the book and see the play and get back to me. I called a month later, she said she would read the book and see the play and get back to me in two weeks. I called two weeks later. She didn't return my call. I called, faxed, etc. She wouldn't even take the time to tell me that she hadn't read the book and seen the play. I still don't know why.

By this time it was May. I realized that despite the fact that I had a copyright, the truth of the matter was that I could not afford a consultation with a lawyer and I didn't want to be lied to again by someone with so-called good intentions. So I came up with a new idea. I would forget about the legal side of this and simply get the story in print. All I had to do was send copies of the book to some theater critics who had already seen the play. They would write about the scandal, and then all the issues of what really happened during the A I D S crisis could surface and everything could get cleared up. Boy, was I dumb.

This is something Don Shewey and I have disagreed about through this whole thing. *Why should anyone care?* Why should anyone be interested that a major blockbuster play about A I D S was stolen from a lesbian on the Lower Eastside? Why should anyone care that what it is saying about the A I D S crisis is false and, at the same time, overshadows what gay men and lesbians have to say about it? And I guess he has a point. I expected people to find this interesting, and really they didn't. Authentic representation of gay and lesbian life is not yet a concern of public discourse.

The first person I sent the materials to was Michiko Kakutani at the *New York Times*. She had just written a full-page column in the Sunday magazine about how loathsome the false bohemia of *Rent* was. Since she'd attacked the falsity of *Rent,* I assumed she would be equally interested in the authentic version. I never heard back.

I can hear Don in my head, "Why should she care?" I really don't have an answer to that question. Because it's true? I guess that in the New York power spectrum some people's lives are more important than others. And while my life and my friends' lives are not the *least* important, they are less important. But I persevered. Actually, given my personality, if the people I contacted had called or written me back with the reasons why they couldn't pursue it, I probably would have given up a lot earlier. But it was all the cold shoulders that kept me going. And also the weird, insulting reactions, like the Midwestern leftie-magazine editor who said I should be "flattered" by the imitation but wouldn't write about it. Or the glossy-magazine editor who said that the influence was obvious but hey, that's post-modernism. These people just revved my motor.

Then I sent the materials to Laurie Stone, a cultural critic at the *Village Voice*. She has always been very supportive of gay and lesbian theater, and she called me back with a very nice message. But she was busy writing two books of her own against deadline and didn't have time to read my novel. She was the first one to decline in a respectful way, and I appreciated it.

I talked the situation over with a few friends of mine who are journalists. My friend Michael Bronski read the book and saw the play and was completely convinced. He pitched the story to *OUT,* the national glossy gay magazine. They turned him down. I ran into Dudley Saunders, the performer whose piece, *Deathblues,* I had loved so much and reviewed the year before. Dudley was writing for *Rolling Stone* magazine and I told him the story. Later that summer Dudley and the novelist Darius James and I were at my birthday party talking about the whole thing. Darius really encouraged Dudley to write something about it. Dudley had already read the book and told me he would go see the play and let me know.

Then I sent the materials to Frank Rich at the *New York Times.* I chose him because he had formerly been the chief theater critic, had been the major champion of *Angels in America,* and was now in this strange position on the op-ed page in relation to gay people. Since the *Times* had never had an openly gay man with his own column, or (God forbid) a gay woman, Rich was the substitute, the resident defender of homosexuals. At the same time he was more progressive on a number of gay-related issues than the narrow cadre of gay conservatives who were allowed to publish in the *Times* on occasion. I was shocked when he actually got back to me. By this point I had been snubbed so many times, I didn't expect anyone at his level to respond. But he wrote me a very nice note asking me to call him in August. I did, but he was at the Democratic Convention. Then I called again in September, and sent a note in October. All this time I was sending updates and faxes and leaving informational messages with my editor, who never responded at all.

Then, in the early fall, I did a benefit reading for Jews for Racial and Economic Justice. One of the other people on the program was Tony Kushner, the author of *Angels in America.* We had met when we were both being arrested for the Irish Lesbian and Gay Organization on Saint Patrick's Day. He had been very helpful to me during the publication of my sixth novel, *Rat Bohemia,* and was always willing to help out. Tony was very familiar with *Rent,* since he had once been asked to direct it. He had also read my book, so those two basic obstacles were already out of the way. Once I laid out all

18

the parallels, without drawing any conclusions himself, he strongly encouraged me to pursue legal action if I believed the work had been plagiarized. He said that writers should protect their work. I was afraid to go through the humiliations again, but he was very inspiring, telling me about the action he had taken when a television movie used ideas from *Angels.*

Around that time the *Wall Street Journal* did a story on Larson's estate. Between licensed productions in major cities around the world, the sale of music rights to David Geffen, the sale of film rights to Robert DeNiro, CDs, videos and a Bloomingdale's franchise of thrift-store style clothing from the play, the Larson estate was now worth one billion dollars. In the middle of the night I suddenly realized that if Larson had done the right thing and taken out an option on my novel, even at the rock bottom rate of 2.5 percent, my share would now be $25 million. I called Tony and told him that I did want to go through with a legal thing. He called a good lawyer that he knew, who we'll call Q.T., and asked him to talk to me on the phone for free. Then I waffled again.

I kept bouncing back and forth in my mind about the question of legal action. I wanted the story to just surface, but it seemed as if without legal action, it never would. On the other hand, I had enormous fears about taking on people at that level of power. They could suck up all my energy, slander me, drag me through the courts for the rest of my life, and ruin my career. And they could pay other people to do all this without having to think twice.

Right around that time, Alisa Solomon, a theater critic for the *Voice,* called me at home. She was doing a story about *Rent*'s dramaturg, Lynn Thompson, suing the estate for a more equitable share than the $2,000 she had been originally paid. Alisa had heard a rumor that I was also suing. It's funny how, along the line, many people have come up to me and told me that they'd heard I was suing. It really goes to show how deceived people are about access to legal justice. They just assumed that I would be able to sue, but the truth was that I did not have enough money to protect my copyright. Yet they all assumed that they, too, would be able to sue in a similar situation. Perhaps this is the result of too many T V programs about lawyers helping poor people get their fair shake. I assured Alisa that I was not suing, but I pointed out other aspects of the situation that might be of equal or even more interest, such as the question of how A I D S is going to be represented in this society. She doubted that she could get anything in without a lawsuit, but that she would try. Then she called me back the night before the piece came out. All the stuff about my situation had been cut by her editor.

This was the beginning of a whole trend. People were interested in whether or not I was suing. Nothing else about the case attracted them. I called Q.T.

"You have a fat-cat defendant here," he said. "Send me all your materials."

So I sent him everything that I knew.

One fall day, soon after, Dudley called me from a pay phone on the street outside the Nederlander Theater on Broadway. He had just seen *Rent* and he was furious. Dudley is the real version of the fake story at the heart of *Rent*. He is an H I V-positive, gay male artist and musician living in the East Village, and he felt violated by what he had just seen on stage. He had also found many more similarities between the play and my novel than I had, and he was determined to get the story out.

In the meantime, the Lynn Thompson story broke, and about a week later, I got a call from Frank Rich of the *New York Times*. He had taken the time to read the book and said that he saw many "similarities." He encouraged me to pursue the case legally. I was deeply appreciative that someone with so much power had taken the time to read my novel and get back to me when he saw the similarities. But he also warned me that the *Times* would not be able to write about these similarities unless there was a lawsuit. They could cover an externally instigated event, but they could not originate the story themselves, regardless of its merit.

Dudley pitched the story to *Rolling Stone.* They turned him down.

I faxed Q.T. about my conversation with Frank Rich. He called me back and told me that he'd reviewed all the materials and felt confident enough to pass them on to his litigating partners. I had made one more step.

Dudley pitched the story to *New York* magazine. Nothing happened. He pitched it to the *Voice.*

"Oh, yeah, we know about that," the editor said and then turned him down.

Dudley had a theory about why everyone was passing on this story. They'd all played such a heavy part in puffing up *Rent,* and they weren't ready to take the heat if it was revealed to be a fraud. The Velvet Mafia were involved, the Glitteratti. *Rent* was glamorous and had social currency, both gay and straight. Everyone wanted to be part of it. The C D had just come out. Soon there would be a celebrity C D, then the film. All these publications wanted cover stories, wanted to be invited to the parties. I was a little nobody. I had no social currency. Why should they alienate *Rent?* There was nothing in it for them.

Patrick Merla, who had been my editor a decade before at the *New York Native,* leaked the story to another department at *New York* magazine. The reporter, a young woman, called me and wanted to know if I was going to sue. No, I told her. But if she would just read the book and see the play . . . It didn't sound like she wanted to have to do anything to get the story. She just wanted the gossip about a lawsuit.

"Do you think I should sue?" I asked her.

"Sure," she said. "You might get some money to keep your mouth shut."

I never heard from her again.

I started to think about money. Money. MONEY. Everyone around me was obsessed with the idea of me getting a sickeningly large amount of money. And many of them, with no experience of real money or of people with real power, believed that I could. I realized something very strange about myself. I have never been a person who really wanted a lot of money. I have never made a decision in my life that was based on money. I have never dreamed of $25 million. A few hundred thousand would be nice. Then I could buy an apartment in an elevator building. But, when I started, for the first time in my life, to think about what I would do with $25 million, $5 million, $1 million, etc.—it all started to get very blurry and vague and scary. What I've always dreamed of and wanted for my life was to have my work be evaluated fairly on the basis of its merit and not be excluded from American literature because of its lesbian content. I've always wanted to be part of American intellectual life and still be able to be completely out of the closet in every way. And this picture, of $25 million, or whatever, did not produce that desired result. I began to be sure that this was not going to end up being about money. That was too simple.

Dudley called me on the phone. He'd been going over the script to *Rent,* and he'd realized something major that fully and completely proved the plagiarism that was already obvious. It had to do with one of the details in *Rent* that was also in my novel: the fact of watch alarms going off in public places to remind men to take their A Z T.

Now, he pointed out, this could not be a coincidence. When I was writing *People in Trouble,* A I D S literature had just barely begun. What existed up to that time was fiction, primarily by people with A I D S or their lovers, dealing with deterioration and death. Books like *Second Son* by Robert Ferro, or memoirs like *Someone Was Here* by George Whitmore, and *Borrowed Time* by Paul Monette, made up the foundations of this new work. But witness fiction had barely emerged. I remember *In Memory of Angel Clare,* by Christopher Bram, as an exception of lasting quality. So *People in Trouble* was among those early pioneers of witness fiction and one of the first to describe A I D S activism. But even this classification is problematic. I'll never forget Michael Bronski's comment at the Key West Writers' Conference that the only reason something exists called "A I D S fiction" is because of homophobia. Otherwise it would be called American fiction. Yet this is the category that we must live with and, therefore, the one I will refer to in this investigation.

Because of this strange situation, writing a novel at the beginning of a new literary class, there was not yet a common language for how to create A I D S fiction. There were no established paradigms, agreed-upon images that could serve as code or shorthand. That was why I'd chosen social realism for the book. I needed a smooth surface texture to explore the complex idea at the root of the novel, namely that personal homophobia becomes societal neglect, that there is a direct relationship between the two. The frameworks were wide open and very unclear.

When I realized that I had no established vocabulary for writing about the epidemic, I made a list of hundreds of details of the A I D S crisis that I observed from my lived experience. Then I selected fifty and used them throughout the novel, hoping that some would resonate broadly and be part of the beginning of a literary A I D S vocabulary. Some of the things I observed and selected did resonate, like watching Rock Hudson on T V as he was being rushed to the airport. Some were quickly outdated and forgotten, like men spreading A L721 on their morning toast. But here was one that seemed to linger; watch alarms going off in public places to remind people to take their A Z T.

As Dudley excitedly pointed out to me, in 1987 when I was writing *People in Trouble,* A Z T was taken every four hours, so people needed watch alarms. But, in 1992 when Larson was writing *Rent,* A Z T was prescribed to be taken every twelve hours, so there would be no watch alarms. It was a detail Larson could only have gotten

23

from one place—my novel. He wouldn't have observed it in 1992, because it was no longer there to observe. And my book was the first place it was ever articulated as a cultural marker.

Dudley went to a different editor at the *Voice* and pitched the story again. This time they said yes. He interviewed the prime players and began to gather even more incriminating information. No one who worked on the project, not Billy Aronson, Larson's original collaborator, nor Michael Greif, the final director, was ever present when Larson just happened to think of any of the material that also appeared in my book. Clearly, Dudley was able to establish that if Larson did coincidentally happen to imagine every idea in my novel, it never happened in front of another human being. Dudley did his research and prepared his story. But the last step was that he had to get a comment from New York Theater Workshop. He called their office and left a message but no one ever called him back. Then he got a phone call from his editor at the *Voice*. New York Theater Workshop had gone over his head, found out who his editor was, and called him. The story was now killed. The official reason? The editor began stuttering in his phone conversation, breaking the news to Dudley. According to the *Voice,* they killed the story because there were many things in my book that did not appear in the play. Huh? That didn't make sense. Dudley argued that the *Voice* had a responsibility to report the issue because it was being widely discussed. But the story was dead.

I called Q.T. What was taking so long? He assured me that his litigating partners had reviewed the materials and had found them compelling enough to move to the next step. They had read the novel and gone to see the play and were now about to write up their report and make a final decision.

I faxed this information to my editor. No answer.

Completely depressed, I called a friend, a straight novelist who has always been there in case of emergency. No matter how desperate the crisis, she always has a clear and coherent suggestion.

She recommended that I talk to a friend of hers who writes for the *Times,* a man we'll call Seymour, who I'd heard of but never met. So, the next day I phoned him at home. When I introduced myself he became immediately upset.

"Oh, no, I absolutely cannot talk to you about this. Oh, no, this is terrible. I'm sorry, no, I can't even discuss it. Good-bye." And he hung up.

About an hour later I called him back.

"Sorry to bother you, Seymour, but you seem absolutely panicked."

"This is terrible, you'll be ruined. If you sue *Rent* you'll be blacklisted from the theater forever. Your career will be ruined. You'll be known forever as the girl who sued *Rent,* and it will eclipse all your other work. And everyone near you will be ruined."

Even though I still hadn't made up my mind, I still had no lawyer, so I assured him that I wasn't suing anyone. Even if I had wanted to I couldn't, because I still didn't have a lawyer. I asked him if there was any other way to get the story out. He said he'd let me know.

Then Dudley called. Finally, he had convinced *New York* magazine to run the story that the *Voice* had killed. I faxed my editor as well as Morticia, the evil junior agent, that the story was about to appear. Neither responded. Then I waited.

ACT TWO

The piece came out in *New York* magazine on January 13, 1997, while I was working at the Key West Literary Seminar, "A I D S and the Literary Imagination." It was a gathering of all the major living practitioners of A I D S literature.

The first call I made was to my editor.

"Oh, has it come out?" she literally yawned. She hadn't even bothered to get it. I suggested she go downstairs to the newsstand in the Saatchi & Saatchi building and buy a copy. The next day I called her back.

"I didn't get any of the faxes or messages that you left with my assistant," she told me. "Anyway, I checked with people around here, and they don't want to sue."

I tried to control my frustration at her laziness and explained quietly that I was not suing. I pointed out that her company owned the rights to a novel that was the unacknowledged source of *Rent,* a huge smash hit that would be in cities all around the world and would soon be a film produced by Robert DeNiro, and that it might be in her company's best interest to let some stores and publications know about this so that they could sell some more books. And that, furthermore, theatrical rights aside, other *Rent* products were being developed and sold, violating Penguin's copyright as well as mine. She yawned a few times more, clearly uninterested.

The conference in Key West is an entirely other story, too complicated to be related in full here. It was tense, difficult, fascinating, with dramatic highs and dramatic lows. For me the most important highs were a brilliant reading by Mark Doty and a very important conversation with the audience about the use of Christian paradigms in understanding A I D S. We talked about why some people need to feel that there is a *reason* that they have A I D S and need to "build a relationship" with their virus. We discussed the ideas/emotional convictions that *suffering makes you better* and the ways in which A I D S has been seen to mitigate homosexuality. It was a conversation that was troublesome, unresolved, and crucial for those of us recording the crisis in literature.

Ironically but predictably, the glossy gay press did not cover this conference, they were too busy interviewing straight icons. But the *New York Times* did send Dinitia Smith to write it up. I had had one interaction with Smith earlier that year. She had written a profile of Sapphire, whose first novel *Push* had just been published by Knopf. Sapphire has been a lesbian literary icon for over twenty years and is at the center of underground lesbian culture. Yet in her piece, Smith buried a statement about how Sapphire *in the seventies experimented with drugs, prostitution, and lesbianism* and never mentioned her homosexuality again, even though it is a pivotal point in Sapphire's literary trajectory. I had a phone conversation the next day with Joan Nestle, the lesbian writer and historian who is a senior member of the community, and we discussed the strange, obliterating experience of seeing twenty years of lesbian history wiped away in that kind of moment of false record. So I was a bit downhearted to see that someone without a clue was the person sent to cover this conference.

I went up to Smith and showed her that week's *New York* magazine article and asked her to include the information in her coverage.

"Oh, no," she said. "You should have come to us first. Now that it has been covered in *New York* we can't mention it."

"But I did go to you first," I said. "I sent it all to Michiko Kakutani in May. I called Seymour. I talked to Frank Rich. He said that the *Times* couldn't initiate coverage, but here someone else has."

"Sorry," she said. "You should have come to us first."

"But I did go to you first."

What I should have done is gone over to Key West's city hall and changed my name to Franz Kafka. But instead, I walked into the auditorium, where a panel on AIDS theater had just broken up and went over to Frank Rich, whom I had never met before.

"Hi, I'm Sarah Schulman," I said, shaking his hand. And I went on this upset rambling jag trying to explain this weird no-win situation that I had found myself in. He was very nice about it but couldn't offer any real solutions.

"What do you want?" asked his wife, Alex Witchel, who had also come down for the conference. "You got the plagiarism story in *New York*."

"I know," I said. "But there are larger issues."

"Like what?" she asked.

"Like how AIDS is going to be represented in this culture."

"That's not news," she said.

When I got home to New York I called Q.T.

"We've read all your materials," he told me. "My litigating partners went to see the play and read the novel, and now we've decided not to represent you."

"Oh," I said, surprise being the furthest thing from my mind. At this point I was chronically numb. I thought I'd heard it all.

"But there is something that I think I should tell you," he said, stammering slightly for the first time in all of our conversations over so many months. "Uhm, well, uh. There is a chance . . . you see . . . well, we've decided to represent the Larson family."

So I decided to write this book. Ask the big questions myself, and then try to answer them. When you're talking about one billion dollars, the water is full of sharks. I realized that I'm too small and they're too big. Maybe that would change someday and I would be able to get legal satisfaction. But, in the meantime, since Larson was dead, there was no one's ego at stake. As long as I didn't ask for money, no one was going to bother me. Now I'd get to the big questions that I've been waiting so long for someone else to ask.

ACT THREE

By the summer of 1997, my inaction was reaching a new level of discomfort. I hadn't found anyone to help me, but I was getting madder and madder about the whole situation. Signs had gone up around my neighborhood in restaurants and cafes saying *"Rent* takes place here." They had started an ad campaign where every ad in an entire subway car was for *Rent.* Many mornings I'd be stuck in the *Rent* car staring at my feet. But most disturbing was the fact that more and more watered-down images and stories about AIDS and homosexuality were worming their way into the culture. The big pro-marriage campaign was well under way. The kitschification of A I D S was at a new height. And everywhere I turned, "normal" homosexuals were given platforms preaching assimilation and, like Andrew Sullivan, claiming that homophobia was no longer an issue. I had spent my entire career facing huge professional obstructions because I refused to repress or code the lesbian content of my work. I had spent years of my life watching gay men die of A I D S while their families and straight society abandoned them. And here, surrounding me on the 6 train, was this glossy billion-dollar lie. The whole thing made me sick. I called a few more lawyers.

I met with a nice woman who works in the same building as Robert DeNiro. Since he owns the film rights to *Rent* we had to whisper in her office. When I told her about Q.T.'s litigating partners reading all my materials and then representing the other side, she was shocked. Apparently that was illegal.

"You should go to the Bar," she said. But she wouldn't take the case. She thought it would overwhelm her practice.

Then a funny thing happened. Lynn Thompson's suit came to trial. Of course, I followed it very closely in the newspapers. Thompson claimed that she had done an extraordinary amount of work on *Rent* and was entitled to more money. Larson's estate, which had been inherited by his parents and sister, had offered a settlement but Thompson wanted more. She had very substantial people testifying on her behalf, including Tony Kushner and Craig Lucas. She also showed very clearly that Larson had no idea of how to write narrative. This really piqued my interest, and I took another look at the specifics of the case.

Thompson had filed a $40-million suit demanding coauthorship and a percentage of the profits. She said she had written 9 percent of the song lyrics and 48 percent of the libretto.

Now, I've never met or spoken to Thompson. I don't know her, but considering my own experience, I took her claims very seriously. After all, Larson had stolen from my book, had acknowledged to other people, like Michael Korie, that he'd used the book, and had never, ever, tried to contact me or work out anything with me. So, I was developing a low opinion of him and believed her claim.

Although the judge acknowledged Thompson's contributions as considerable, she lost the case. One of the dramatic courtroom moments that the *Times* reported was that the family's lawyer (ironically, the people who had reviewed all of my materials) asked her to recite one of the lyrics from the show, and she couldn't remember it. I was completely sympathetic. The courts just don't understand what art-making is like. Artists make so many things and work on so many projects and have so many characters and words and plots in their heads, they just can't always remember all of it right away. Many times, readers have asked me a question about some character or plot point and I can't precisely recall it. There are just too many ideas to all sit on the mind's shelf. But the legal system doesn't understand how the creative mind works, and so Thompson got screwed.

However, of even more interest to me was all the evidence she introduced to show that Larson couldn't write plot, something that many people had mentioned to me as I was gathering information. This seemed obvious, considering that the straight plot of *Rent* was a rehash of *La Bohème*. Between *People in Trouble* and *La Bohème* it was almost all adaptation. But here, in Thompson's case, were the particulars. Before *Rent,* Larson had few credits to his name. He had written songs for *Sesame Street, Superbia* at Playwrights Horizons, and a one-man show, *Tick, Tick . . . BOOM.* But he had never written a full book for a musical, and never written anything complex with multiple characters. When he first brought *Rent* to New York Theater Workshop, they advised him to hire a librettist to write the musical's book.

"When I got it, it had no coherent structure," Thompson said.

"Jonathan was a genius as a composer, but he had a lot of limitations as a playwright."

At this point I started to get mad again and went back to pursuing lawyers. Urvashi Vaid, the gay organizer, referred me to a lawyer. A friend of mine, an artist who had had a video piece stolen by Gucci, referred me to the same lawyer. I sent him all my materials. Then he referred me to another lawyer at a large arts firm. She responded immediately. That was a switch.

In the meantime, my publisher had refused to do any publicity for the *New York* magazine piece. After a lot of effort on my part, they finally agreed to fax the article to a list I had given them, but I had to call them three times about it before the fax even went out, and there was no follow-up. Yet the grassroots gay press started to report the story. Little pieces appeared in *Lambda Book Report, Harvard Gay and Lesbian Review,* and *Feminist Bookstore News.* Michael Bronski interviewed me on all the far-ranging questions of the case for *Gay Community News.* The *Minneapolis City Paper* did a story to accompany the Minneapolis opening of *Rent.* The London *Gay Times* did a piece. I was writing book reviews for *The Advocate* at the time and sent them all the clips, but I was told that one of the editors was a friend of Larson's and so they wouldn't be reporting the story.

Then Laurie Wiener did a piece on the case for a gay paper, *Chicago Outlines,* in which she interviewed a vice president for legal affairs at Penguin about why they had taken no action on my behalf. This had continued to be a big mystery. I did not understand why Penguin didn't pursue the matter legally, especially now that CDS, books, and other products beyond the scope of theater were on the market. I certainly did not understand why they didn't publicize the issue, even without legal action, simply to get more copies of the novel out there. A Penguin spokesman told Wiener that Penguin could have a legal interest, even though I had retained theatrical rights, because the publisher does typically carry a "variable legal interest" in derivative works. So, there were grounds for Penguin to act! More to the point, he had never actually heard of this case, which made me wonder how much investigating my editor had actually done within the company. I began to wonder if she had just stonewalled the whole thing. While this information opened up the possibility for legal action on Penguin's part, it still did not explain why they would not publicize.

Then I got a phone call from Achy Obejas at the *Chicago Tribune*. *Rent* was about to open in Chicago, she had read the story in *Chicago Outlines* and wanted to see my materials. I sent them right away. I was still talking to the lawyers who had finally responded, Christine LePera, Jane Simon, and Michael Emanuelian from Gold, Farrell & Marks. Even though they assured me in plain English that they knew that Larson had "used" my book, I had been so humiliated by all my previous lawyer encounters that I didn't really think they would follow-up. But my cynicism turned out to be misplaced, and they went around doing research, conducting interviews, and developing a legal theory, building a case.

Achy did a great job researching the story. She reviewed all my evidence and found that everything I was saying was accurate. But she went even farther. Picking up on Dudley's idea, she interviewed a wide range of Larson's collaborators, from Billy Aronson, his original partner, to Lynn Thompson, his final collaborator. None of them claimed to have either thought of or witnessed the introduction of any of the material that was duplicated from my novel. This was extraordinary evidence. A piece of musical theater is a highly collaborative product. It takes years in development with readings, workshops, and endless rewrites. It is highly unusual that the core plot, characterizations, and dynamics of a piece would have been developed in isolation. Yet no one remembered Larson saying "I know, let's make her a performance artist." Or, "I know, how about something about watch alarms?" Especially for someone like Larson, who was known to not be able to write narrative.

As her enquiry progressed, it became even more apparent that the main narrative material that Larson brought into the collaboration was from *People in Trouble*.

Interestingly, when Achy interviewed the attorney for the Larson family, Owen Snyder, he claimed in print that he had never heard of me. But this was impossible. Remember, his firm had reviewed my materials for three months. Two days later, I got a letter from Q.T. In it was a fax he'd received from Snyder claiming that he'd forgotten that he'd seen my papers. Clearly they were worried about the conflict of interest, and I guessed that their clients, the Larson family, probably didn't know that the law firm they were paying a lot of money to was actually disqualified from any litigation involving me. It was a royal fuck-up on their part, and just the mistake that might make things easier for my case.

That was the final straw, two weeks before Thanksgiving 1997. Gold, Farrell & Marks sent a letter to the Larson family, telling them that they had infringed my work. They also sent a letter to the Larsons' attorney informing him that he was disqualified from representing the family in any proceeding involving me.

Fairly quickly, we received a reply from Larson's father, Allen. In one way he was very rude and blustery to the attorney, but he also described himself as "open-minded" and willing to look at the evidence. Although he said he would not purchase *People in Trouble,* he did invite us to send him a copy. Here are excerpts from the letter we sent him, which I think is worth reproducing because it is the final summation of our argument as the Larson Estate heard it.

December 3, 1997

Dear Mr. Larson,

. . . You have asked for a copy of *People In Trouble* and we enclose two copies of the work herewith. In addition, we set forth below a summary of some of the factors which have led us to conclude that Mr. Larson not only had access to *People In Trouble,* but that he used significant material from

33

the work in creating *Rent*. We believe that if you truly approach this matter with an open mind, you will reach the same conclusion as we.

First, it is important that you know something about our client, Sarah Schulman. Ms. Schulman is a widely respected chronicler of gay and lesbian life, the East Village and the A I D S crisis. She was a member of Act Up for seven years. *People In Trouble* was her fourth out of nine published works, four of which deal with the A I D S crisis. Eight of her books are set in the East Village, including *People In Trouble*. Among her many awards she has received a 1984 Fulbright Fellowship in Judaic Studies, residencies at McDowell and Yaddo, two New York Foundation for the Arts Fiction Fellowships, and Gustavus Meyers Book Award for Promoting Social Tolerance. Ms. Schulman is currently a Visiting Writer at Barnard College. In 1993, she was a Regent's Fellow in Judaic Studies at the University of California at Santa Cruz. This Spring she will be a Writer-In-Residence University of California at San Diego. She was awarded a 1997 Stonewall Award for "improving the lives of gays and lesbians in the United States," and was a 1997 finalist for the Prize de Rome. In short, Ms. Schulman is an established, respected and serious author who has interposed this claim only after careful consideration.

People In Trouble was written by Ms. Schulman in 1987–88. It was published by Dutton in 1990. A paperback edition was published by Plume/ New American Library in 1991. The book was awarded The Words Project for A I D S Prize for Fiction in 1991. *People In Trouble* was nominated for a Lambda Literary Award. The book has been translated into German, Swedish, Spanish and published in British edition. It was favorably reviewed in *The New York Times, The Nation, The Village Voice, The San Francisco Chronicle, The Guardian of London* and a number of other significant review venues. It has sold approximately 25,000 copies.

People In Trouble is set in the late 1980's East Village and focuses on artists, the homeless, gays and lesbians and people with A I D S. The intermingling of these people and social conditions provides the backdrop of the novel. In the foreground is a triangular love relationship. Kate, a selfish artist, is ending a relationship with a male artist, Peter, and beginning an affair with a lesbian, Molly, a social activist. However, she is conflicted about her new sexual identity and continues to flirt with Peter. There is a sub-plot about an inter-racial gay male couple, one of whom is a drag queen, and one of whom has A I D S. The death of the drag queen is a cathartic moment in the dramatic structure of the novel. Inspired by him and his suffering, Kate produces a work of performance art designed to neutralize the greedy landlord who is evicting people with A I D S. The exhibition of this work is also a major dramatic moment in the novel's structure. In *People In Trouble,* the surviving gay lover, a Black man, is an activist for the poor and HIV-infected. He and his friends organize a scheme using credit cards at a grocery store to feed the hungry.

Rent similarly is set in the East Village and concerns artists, the homeless, gays and lesbians and people with A I D S. *Rent* also has a pivotal triangular love relationship. Maureen, a performance artist, has recently broken up with Mark, a filmmaker, and is beginning an affair with a lesbian, Joanne, a social activist. Maureen continues to flirt with Mark. As the play progresses, Maureen produces a work of performance art designed to neutralize the greedy landlord who is evicting people with A I D S. Her performance of this work is a major dramatic moment in the play's structure. Two other dominant characters in *Rent* parallel those in *People In Trouble* and the events which affect their lives: Angel, a drag queen, is involved in an inter-racial affair with Tom Collins. Both have A I D S. Angel's death is a cathartic moment in the dramatic structure of the play. Tom, who is Black, rewires a cash machine at a grocery store to help feed the poor.

A difference between *Rent* and *People In Trouble* only serves to highlight the use of our client's work in the creation of the later work. Thus, *Rent* is set in the 1990s, rather than the late 1980's. However, anachronistically, the use of watch alarms to remind people with A I D S to take their medications is a prominent paradigm. When Sarah Schulman was writing *People In Trouble,* in 1987, A Z T was prescribed to be taken every four hours, necessitating the use of watch alarms, which would then go off in public places where there were many people with A I D S, such as the Act Up meetings that she attended every Monday night. Her use of this image in *People In Trouble* is the first articulated observation of this cultural detail. In the 1990's, when Mr. Larson was writing and setting *Rent,* A Z T was prescribed every twelve hours, so no one would have been using watch alarms. Mr. Larson could not have observed this detail at that time, because it was not there to be observed.

There is no need to rely on these striking similarities or, indeed on the dissemination of *People In Trouble,* to place the work in Mr. Larson's hands. In 1987, while writing *People In Trouble,* Sarah met Stewart Wallace and Michael Korie, an operatic team who wanted to make the novel into an opera. The three developed a treatment which circulated for the next three years to many prominent houses in the US and Europe including the Public Theater, Brooklyn Academy of Music and Lincoln Center. The package included the treatment and various drafts of the manuscript, finally including the published book once it appeared in 1990. They alternatively described their project as "a *La Boheme* for the '90s" or "a *Westside Story* for the '90s." Among those approached with this project was Ira Weitzman, whom the official *Rent* book advises ultimately suggested to Billy Aronson that he collaborate with Jonathan Larson.

Moreover, in 1994, Michael Korie and Jonathan Larson were both awarded a Richard Rodgers Prize and both attended the awards dinner. At the dinner, Mr. Larson described the plot of his play to Mr Korie who responded "That sounds like *People In Trouble* by Sarah Schulman." Mr. Larson expressed surprise that Mr. Korie was aware of the novel and affirmed that he had read the book and was using it in creating *Rent.*

Finally, Billy Aronson has repeatedly stated that when he was working with Jonathan Larson on a collaboration that would come to be *Rent,* none of the content that overlaps with *People In Trouble* was in the project. Aronson says that the material came in once Jonathan went off to work on his own. Concomitantly, both Michael Greif and Lynn Thompson say that the overlapping materials were already in place when they came into the project. This leaves, as we stated in our initial letter, the inclusion of the infringing material in the hands of Larson.

36

The official *Rent* book freely admits that Mr. Larson was not adept at writing complex narrative or developing plot lines. There are only two basic plot lines in *Rent: People In Trouble* and *La Boheme*. Ms. Schulman should be compensated for the use of her material.

Then we waited for a response from the estate. It came about three weeks later on December 29, 1997, from a new and different law firm. So, I guessed that their lawyers did accept that there was a conflict of interest after all.

They stated very firmly that "RENT is an original work by Jonathan Larson." They said that "we do not believe that the alleged similarities, to the extent that there are any, are anything more than coincidental." Their letter was very interesting to me because they claimed coincidences when clearly there was too much overlap for that to be possible. But their claim was vague. They just said the word "coincidental," they did not refute a single point in my letter nor did they give any explanations other than mine. Their focus, instead, was on copyright law. "Your client's claim, at best, is based upon ideas, as opposed to the expression of ideas. Copyright does not extend to the 'building blocks of creative expression' which typically include, among other things, the work's theme, plot and stock characters and settings."

This statement from them really validated my position. Perhaps not in the Legal World, but certainly in the Human World. For even if, as they claimed, the similarities were not actionable legally because he didn't use my exact words, the fact that he used my "theme, plot and stock characters and settings" was enough for me. I didn't need it to correspond to the technicalities of the law, it just is plainly obvious for anyone to see—the "building blocks" of *Rent* came from my novel.

Besides, I agree with his lawyers that he used my ideas, not the "expression" of my ideas. In fact, he used my ideas to express something that is the opposite of what I expressed. It may not be legally binding, but it is immoral, especially given the meaning of my novel versus the meaning of his play.

Since I felt validated humanly, at the same time that I was convinced I could not win legally, I decided not to pursue the matter through the courts. And, in all ways this outcome was a huge relief. As I've said before, I was very afraid of going through a legal process against such a powerful corporate entity and their social currency. I feared that my life would be ruined. So, actually, this result, ending legal approaches but validating my position morally, was in my personal best interest. Once I accepted this, I realized that I was now freed to go on to the larger questions that had always been at the root of this matter, namely the *meaning* of this situation. How could a nation devastated by the AIDS crisis embrace a popular cultural "expression" that distorted the reality of that crisis? This is a contradiction that I will attempt to analyze in the two following sections of this book.

SIMULACRA,

AUTHENTICITY, AND THE

THEATRICAL CONTEXT

OF <u>RENT</u>

PART 2

I have the pleasure and the privilege of writing part of this book at an arts colony in a quiet, subsidized studio surrounded by deer, wild turkeys, and fiddlehead ferns. Time alone in the country can be illuminating for a city girl, and over the weeks that I've been here I've had to face a very harsh fact about my life. I am a relic of a disappeared civilization.

When I first had the opportunity to come to this wonderful retreat eleven years ago, I was working as a waitress at Leroy's Coffee Shop in Tribeca. I had finished my second novel for Seal Press, a feminist publisher based in Seattle, Washington. But, I had never had an in-depth discussion with another novelist. I really didn't know any. Coming to this colony changed my life forever for the better. I met and made friends with artists I love and respect. I was exposed to ideas about art and culture that I had never heard before. These were oppositional ideas, not official ideas. That's why I'd never heard them before. For example, that initial visit in 1986 was the first time I'd ever heard that a life that does not follow a conventional narrative like Romance, Marriage, and Motherhood would have a different relationship to a conventional narrative form than one that did. I had written two novels with primary lesbian content, struggling for structure, and not knowing why. This information has permanently deepened my understanding of the world.

Almost all the writers I met in residence in 1986 were independent artists. We had each sat alone in our apartments and written our books according to the rhythm and measure of our own hearts.

We had learned to write by writing. We had amassed eclectic arrays of information by encountering different kinds of books in different ways along our dramatically different lives. When we finished writing our books, we learned about publishing by getting them published. Almost all work-related table conversation was about the art process, art ideas. They were examples of the individual spirit, the discovery and the personal creation of each one's unique, invented writing experience.

At that time I lived in and was documenting life in the East Village. I can't really summarize for you now what life in the East Village was like then, but it is thoroughly documented in my first six novels, which detail the neighborhood from the years 1981 to 1995. Suffice it to say that the East Village was a center for the production of global ideas. It was filled with varied races of immigrants, homosexuals, working people, bohemians, and artists working in both traditional and emerging forms, most of whom had no institutional training or support. It feels strange to say this at age thirty-eight, because it is a statement that should only come from the mouth of someone much older, but that was a civilization that has disappeared. It was destroyed by AIDS, gentrification, and marketing. Now the East Village is primarily a center of consumption for the wealthy.

I recently saw a film by the photographer Nan Goldin, called *I'll Be Your Mirror*. In it she displays the breadth of loss of her friends to AIDS. She is a little older and more successful than I am and moved in a different circle, but it was part of the same extended art world and some of her dead overlapped with mine. I started crying in the theater, because she had spelled out for me the reasons behind the barrenness and loneliness I had begun to feel in my own neighborhood. Afterward, I went up to her and asked for help on how to think about the future. What was our future?

"There aren't many of us left," she said. "That world is over forever."

I felt that she was doing me a favor by telling me this truth. But where do I belong, now?

I come back to this retreat in 1997 filled with gratitude for the extraordinary opportunity. And I do really good work here that I would never have been able to do at home. Yet some things have changed dramatically. Now, almost all of the writers here are graduates of MFA programs. They are more demographically and aesthetically homogenous. Their tabletop conversation is about the famous writers they've gotten recommendations from because they've had them as teachers. They talk about which agents they want, what connections they got through their schools, *The New Yorker,* the hot, straight, white male writers of the moment, publishing, the many fellowships they've accrued. None of them has published or even completed a book. I feel sick.

To be a writer, I guess, now means to enroll in a master's program, workshop your material, be exposed to your professor's reading list and gossip, and be fed into art colonies, publishing houses, agencies, jobs, cliques, and grants. In other words, it is about paying a bribe (tuition) to get contacts with your teachers. How can this possibly be good? Shouldn't an artist create out of a singular vision, resistent to the pressure of group standards? Isn't the world a better place to develop a singular voice than an institution? And why should only the people who have the time or money to go to these programs be the ones who get the advantages? Aesthetically, financially, and spiritually, the whole system seems wrong. And yet, from my point of view as a mid-career writer, these programs are the only way that people like me can earn a living. I know I'm a good teacher, but I hate the snobbish, market-oriented culture of mediocrity these programs are creating. I feel surrounded by its consequences. Yet, given the current financial reality of low advances and no arts funding, MFA programs are the major source of employment for writers in America today. It's a sad narrative arc from WPA to NEA to MFA, but those teaching jobs are the only way many of us can afford to keep writing. So, I focus on the microcosm of the classroom, treat each student individually, do a good job. So many independent artists share these same feelings in private but are afraid to discuss them publicly, for fear of being blacklisted from future employment. It's just like everything else, but much more ironic when applied to art-making, which needs the opposite social condition of individualism and eccentricity to flourish.

In the evenings, here in the country, I have many heated discussions about these questions. I find the topic unavoidable, because the culture of these programs oppressively pervades too many moments. Connections are bragged about, and they're often the same ones. The discoveries of postmodernism, Marxism, and liberation politics are virtually unknown. The MFA students, most of whom are dominant-culture, have no mechanism for seeing how their dominance is constructed; their sense of entitlement and superiority has been reinforced by this disembodied ticket to the publishing industry. Over and over, I hear a defensive, alienating insistence on their sense of their own normalcy and the rightness of their feelings of objectivity.

At first I think that this phenomenon is something like the Victorian aristocrats who hired artists to teach them how to play the piano and paint landscapes. But later I realize that this is the manifestation of the idea of Writing as a Profession instead of as an art form.

This contrast between value systems exactly mirrors my experience with *Rent:* Official Art versus Art. It illuminates for me the appeal of the falsity of *Rent:* how audiences could respond to these artificial ideas about art, about homosexuality, about the East Village. *Rent,* like MFA programs, reflects the power of institutions to normalize privilege, to homogenize aesthetics. The extreme vulnerability of independent artists has broader ramifications for the larger culture. I see it as a shift in public discussion from expression to product. And I extend this understanding to what has happened to my neighborhood. It has been transformed from neighborhood as community, as an interdependent, lived relationship, into neighborhood as museum, as playground, as status symbol. The whole dominant culture has become more conservative and relies on a kind of simulacrum to sustain itself. This commitment to artifice is at the heart of the phenomenon of *Rent.*

One of the most frequent comments I've heard about *Rent*'s representation of artists, gay people, people of color, people with AIDS, homeless people, and so on, is that misrepresentation is a standard bearer of theater. "That's entertainment." From my point of view, that statement is neither acceptable nor true. Of course, the people in power are always telling you that their privileges are a neutral, unavoidable consequence of a natural order. As Audre Lorde, my professor at Hunter College, told our class in 1982, "That you can't fight City Hall is a rumor being spread by City Hall." But, specifically, in 1996, the year that *Rent* opened and was praised in New York City, there were many plays with far more complex and accurate representations of the kinds of people that are used as mere props in *Rent.* These other works were often written by the very people depicted and included complex human beings, instead of signifiers of the audience's tolerance. That year there were plays that were by black women, by lesbians, by gay men; there were important works of art about AIDS, in particular, and the historic burden of morality in general. None of these works received the kind of praise that *Rent* received.

It is not helpful to simply say there were great plays from the margins in the time of *Rent,* because that wouldn't convey their variety, complexity, and humanity. Moreover, these works will have effectively been replaced by *Rent* in the official memory. I want to document here, for once, the actual content of these theatrical expressions during the 1995–96 season so that when I say the "context" of *Rent,* you'll have some inkling of what I mean. It is an excavation of the kind of art work that always goes on but is usually buried either by being ignored or by being antithetically described.

Now I am not a biological determinist, and I do not believe that human beings are incapable of writing authentically about people with less social currency than themselves. As an artist, I want to successfully reveal a broad range of characters, and, as a lesbian, I want to be complexly depicted in the work of others. But, in the spring of 1997 as I am writing this book, every play on a prominent mainstage in New York City that is about homosexuality or A I D S was written by a heterosexual (*A Question of Mercy* by David Rabe, *The Young Man from Atlanta* by Horton Foote, *One Flea Spare* by Naomi Wallace, *Rent* by Jonathan Larson, and *Victor/Victoria* by Blake Edwards). There is nothing inherently wrong with that, but it is a curious fact that has meaning, even on the surface.

It seems as though the post–*Angels in America* theatrical condition is a profoundly retrograde one. Because homosexuality and A I D S have been normalized as the province of heterosexual writers, gay writers are pressured back into metaphor, euphemism, and code. In other words, straight writers can now use A I D S and homosexuality to assert their universality while gay writers must obscure the same subjects to ensure theirs. That is not equality.

Rent opened at New York Theater Workshop on February 22, 1996. That year I was employed as a theater critic for the *New York Press*. My dear friend and critical mentor, Don Shewey, and I wrote a he said/she said column for the free weekly paper. Once or twice a week we would go to the theater together and then write companion columns about how we each experienced the play. At that point I had been a playwright for about fifteen years, but, like most artists in this city, I could rarely go see my own art form performed because of the prohibitive cost of tickets. Don, on the other hand, is a highly respected theater writer. As former theater editor for the *Soho Weekly News* and a longtime contributor to the *Village Voice,* the *New York Times* Arts and Leisure section and *American Theater* magazine, Don has a lifetime of intense theater-going behind him. He is highly knowledgeable about the art of theater criticism and very respectful of the artists. He and I had a contentious friendship for years that often erupted in screaming matches about such topics as the men's movement, among other things, but we really enjoyed arguing with each other. Finally we decided to argue in print.

Our column began in *LGNY,* the local gay newspaper, but after a while we wanted a larger readership, so Don sent our clippings off to *New York Press.* The *Press,* a right-wing alternative to the liberal *Village Voice,* was known for editorials against homeless people and had supported Steve Forbes for president. But I really wasn't prepared for our first meeting with the editorial staff. We were ushered into their executive offices at the prestigious Puck Building in Soho only to discover that we were about to write for a paper with no women, no out queers, and no Blacks, Asians, or Latinos in high editorial positions. Instead we sat stiffly with three dudes while they talked to Don and ignored me. Frankly, I didn't have much to say. Everyone knows the only good thing about the *Press* was its horoscope. I'd never been able to actually read the paper because they never covered anything I was interested in. I just wanted a place to write. The feeling was mutual. The dudes put their cards on the table. They had no gay coverage, no theater, and no sports, they explained. So, with our column they could have queer and theater, which would kill two birds with one stone. Now they just need someone to do sports.

We told them that we wanted to write about theater from a gay perspective, and they nodded their heads in agreement. But it was clear at the start that they had no idea of exactly what that meant. In fact, even I didn't fully understand what that meant until well into the project. Some things were certain from the beginning. We weren't going to closet our reactions as most gay theater critics do. We also would not closet the gay backstage, the queer personalities, sensibilities, and histories that converge on most New York theatrical productions. And, of course, we were not going to pretend that a heterosexual perspective was a neutral, universal one. This last point was the most complex and is something I'm still grappling with.

For example, I recently attended a reading of a workshop for writers facing terminal illnesses, mostly cancer or AIDS. As the evening unfolded, it became increasingly obvious that the straight women with breast cancer and the gay women with breast cancer had divergent concerns. The straight women repeatedly expressed fears that they were losing their femininity or their sexuality. They were afraid that husbands/boyfriends would abandon them post-mastectomy. A number had stories of men who had done exactly that. Some feared never being able to attract a man again. The lesbians, on the other hand, were primarily concerned with death. They did not associate mastectomy with loss of femininity or sexuality and did not express primary fears about being abandoned by their lover or about losing their ability to attract another.

I thought about this event later the same month when I saw Naomi Wallace's play *One Flea Spare* at the Public Theater. One of the assumptions of the play, set in London at the time of the plague, was that Darcy Snellgrave (Dianne Wiest) was starved for physical affection because her husband had refused to touch her body ever since it was scarred in a fire thirty years before. The play was predicated on the audience's understanding his repulsion as reasonable, or at least as a given. The fact of it was not the emotional plot point, Darcy's reaction being given more dramatic weight. I asked myself the meaning of the author's expectations of audience reaction to this information. Given the divergence of attitudes in the illness workshop, I concluded that to accept Wallace's positioning was to view the play from a heterosexual perspective; to problematize it was to view it from a lesbian perspective. What's a critic to do? Do you assume a perspective that is not your own simply because it is a dominant paradigm? That seems to be how most gay theater critics act today. Or do you put it into the context of Lani Guanier's theory of the "Tyranny of the Majority" and assert that a minority opinion can be, indeed that it must be, presented in a normalizing way in order to have a functional democracy. Even in the theater.

The more comfortable I became with these notions, the more complex and, I think, valuable my own theatrical criticism became. Certainly, I had the best possible education, in that Don and I furiously debated all the plays we saw, with all their theatrical, political, and sexual implications. The key to the kingdom of free tickets to anything I wanted to see on the New York stage for nine months helped me articulate a more sophisticated understanding of how false the prevailing illusion of cultural objectivity was. Let's face it, I was extremely lucky to have the opportunity to see this vast range of inspiring work. I got to have a lot of pleasure, and I got to see many artists seriously grappling with the full range of human experience. It was a utopian existence. But, more important to the project of this book, it allowed me to thoroughly explore the theatrical context in which the musical *Rent* emerged.

AIDS AND THE THEATRICAL CONTEXT OF RENT

I guess the most important AIDS precursor to *Rent* was Jonathan Demme's Oscar-winning film *Philadelphia. Philadelphia* stands alone as an example of heterosexual conceit and disregard for truth. The film has been discussed extensively in other places, but, in brief, *Philadelphia* is predicated on the idea that there is no gay community. A gay lawyer (Tom Hanks) has AIDS and is fired by his homophobic law firm. He goes to a straight homophobic lawyer (Denzel Washington) because there are no gay lawyers. It is shocking that an entire film could be built on this premise, which is not only absurd but grossly ahistorical, since the abandonment of people with AIDS by heterosexual society is the most historically significant factor in the initial escalation of the crisis in the United States. Despite this, gay people built a world of services, advocacy organizations, and personal relationships in response to the epidemic that later became the foundation of support for HIV-infected heterosexuals. Gay lawyers were among the first professional sectors to respond to the epidemic. In other words, not only was the premise of *Philadelphia* false, it was the opposite of the actual truth. Yet this film was highly rewarded and made huge moral claims. Throughout the film, gay people are vulnerable, weak, and alone. We take a back seat while the heroic straight people protect us and defend us. In the end of the film, Hanks dies happy.

In many ways *Philadelphia* established a precedent, reinforced by *Rent,* and began the process in which gay-made work about AIDS was pushed to the margins and straight-made work was substituted in its stead. The fact that the screenwriter of *Philadelphia* was gay (a point the makers used over and over again to justify themselves) is irrelevant. After all, Clarence Thomas is black. Still, in the era of *Philadelphia* and *Rent,* it was basically straight-made homosexuality for predominantly straight audiences. In fact it is interesting to note how much permission and territory for work about the heterosexual heroes of AIDS has been grabbed in the short time between the opening of Pulitzer Prize–winner *Rent* and the opening, a year later, of David Rabe's Pulitzer Prize–nominated *A Question of Mercy,* which also premiered at New York Theater Workshop. Rabe's play is about a gay male couple in 1990 in New York City, one of whom is dying of AIDS. They know no gay doctors and have no community of people with AIDS, so they must find a straight doctor to heroically help them with an assisted suicide.

The play makes it clear that the two men do not have sex. This serves two interesting functions. First, it removes the stigma of homosexual sex, thereby rendering the men more palatable to a broad audience. This follows the general trend of AIDS being seen as a mitigating force on homosexuality, something that makes gay people acceptable. As Gabriel Rotello has noted, men who were kicked out of their families for being gay are sometimes allowed back in on the condition that they are dying. Second, the removal of a sexual relationship signals to the ignorant heterosexual audience member that the surviving partner is not at risk and that his possible infection should not be a subtext of the plot. This coding system relies on a heterosexual audience who view a gay male couple on the heterosexual model, assuming that the infected partner got "it" by violating the monogamy norm.

The surviving partner is depicted as weak and fearful. The doctor, a stranger, becomes instantly closer to the dying man than the patient is to his own lover. The three of them decide that the doctor will be with the dying man in his last moments while the lover goes to the movies with his decontextualized heterosexual "best" female friend. Can you imagine a play in which a man goes to the movies while a strange doctor shared his beloved wife's last moments? This plot twist alone reveals the depth of the author's belief in the supremacy of heterosexual relationships over homosexual ones and his unconscious determination to diminish the gay relationship in order to be able to construct these fantasy dynamics in his play.

For the record, I find the reflective, "best"–female friend character (a.k.a. "fag hag") to be a profoundly annoying mainstay of gay male artwork, and it is upsetting to see it picked up in a heterosexual man's play about gay life. But in a way, her presence reveals that the piece is written more from other representations of AIDS and gay life than from lived experience. Because in the real world, unlike in most work by and about gay men, a heterosexual woman who is a close friend of a gay man also has a life of her own.

At the last moment, the morally weak surviving lover betrays his boyfriend's wishes and forces the doctor to break his promise to the patient. Not only does the surviving lover become the catalyst for the doctor's moral flaw, in an updated version of the treacherous homosexual, but his actions actually cause his lover to suffer an unnecessarily agonizing and brutal death, one even worse than he would have suffered had he died of AIDS and not a botched suicide attempt. Once again, straight people are the heroes of AIDS, gay people are weak, vulnerable, morally questionable, and alone.

In the 1995–96 season, when *Rent* opened, there were still a few works being performed that directly addressed AIDS from a truthful, historical, and emotionally authentic perspective. And they were created either by people with AIDS or by participant witnesses. Two outstanding examples of artists who made work about AIDS at the time of *Rent*'s opening were Dudley Saunders and Diamanda Galás.

A few years before these events, I had seen *Birdbones,* a brilliant solo piece by Dudley Saunders, at the Kitchen. It had a virtuosic level of writing, something often missing in performance art. In the summer of 1995, Don and I went to review Dudley's new show at Dixon Place on the Bowery. (Dixon Place originated in the living room of Ellie Covan, a former actor who was known primarily for her work as Jane Bowles, whom she somewhat resembles. After a number of years she moved her living room to a Bowery loft and brought Dixon Place along with it.) The night we saw Dudley's new work, *Deathblues,* I believe there were five people in the audience: a white gay couple, a black leatherman, Don, and me.

Dudley is a studly, long-haired performer with a Kentucky twang and a slight lisp. In *Deathblues* he appears alone, barefoot, and shirtless in overalls, one suspender down to reveal a pierced nipple. A gay spin on the hillbilly aesthetic. He just stood before us and sang. There was no dialogue. He has a gorgeous, intoxicating voice and the musical idioms he'd chosen for that evening were familiar, rich with country and gospel. But, from the first piece, in which a young man stands on a pier, listening to the advice and stories of his grandfather, we realize that all the songs are about AIDS. His grandfather is another gay man, slightly older and aged by disease. The Westside Highway by the Hudson River stands in for the backdrop of rolling hills.

We saw *Deathblues* at a moment in which gay male artists were backing away from A I D S as a subject matter. No one seemed to be interested on the consumer end. The audiences who needed to know didn't want to know, and the ones who did know knew all too well. Art about A I D S in the fall of 1996 was reploughing some established territory while the more ambitious artists moved increasingly into the safer metaphoric range. We were seeing more work about plagues, about other illnesses, about other people (mostly women) with metaphoric diseases, mostly cancer. But I was so fulfilled by what Dudley was able to achieve by taking a chance with truth. At the end of the evening bringing together "T-cells and T-birds" he managed to place A I D S firmly in the context of national folklore by applying it gracefully, with deep emotional resonance, to our most American musical forms. Too bad nobody saw it. Little did I realize at the time how much Dudley's integrity about A I D S would later play a role in the *Rent* scandal.

Diamanda Galás performed her new piece *Schrei X* in January 1996 at Performance Space 122 in a barely perceptible half-light. Her white flesh hovered between a silvery glow and the engulfing darkness. Her long hair and sleeveless black dress disappeared into the night. The piece began with a preparatory silence, loaded and tense. She'd already conveyed the taut preoccupation of her music before the first sound.

When Galás did begin, it was with the power of both breath and breadth, sure enough to fill the room and hearts of the listeners. The high pitch of that first note would normally signify a shriek, an ear-splitting howl. But the absolute skill and control at the root of her music turned this offering far away from clichéd invasion or anticipated assault. It was revealed, instead, to be a song. Galás is emotionally free in her music, but she is also intellectually and formally precise. Her work starts with content, its soul being her absolute refusal ever to give up being devastated by loss. Never to accept unnecessary loss. To refuse to comply with the ever-backsliding definition of acceptability. *Schrei X* is rooted in this explicit statement, but the emotional meaning is conveyed fully through the *expression* of the content. The piece had words but they were anchors, not the foregrounded conveyors of meaning.

Watching an artist of this level of achievement is humbling in a number of ways. First, it is clear that a woman artist of such singular purpose, who has used her smarts in pursuit of her own concerns, has paid a very high personal price. Galás is a survivor. She has refused to allow anyone to stop her, to tell her what to do with her work. The death of her brother Philip Dimitri Galás from AIDS over a decade ago, sparked a visceral and insistent musical and personal confrontation with the disease. Instead of moving on to euphemism, as so many artists have done, she has expanded her emotional understanding to a larger question of confinement, isolation, and the diminishment of status. She has battled to be able to articulate a moral responsibility through her music. And the commitment is long-standing. At the same time her composition is enormously generous. *Schrei X* was the rare kind of work in which an artist investigates an emotion, a condition far too implicating and disquieting for most civilians. And, in the process of this, she comes to a place of enlightenment. The performance was a recounting of what it took and offered us the transformations this work requires. It is the rarest and most crucial path, to commit to more feeling, stronger individuality, and more truthful expression. This is especially true in our culture, where television is increasingly the principle cultural referent, even in metaphoric work about AIDS.

Rent, in addition to its positioning of heterosexuals front and center of the crisis, and its callous privileging of straight people with AIDS over gay people with AIDS, specifically denies the actual AIDS experience, both individually and socially. None of its characters suffers the specific pains or troubles of people with AIDS. The one death is a cinematic death. On the other hand, both Galás and Saunders focus on pain and its costs and on making it undeniable and inescapable for the audience, as it is for people with AIDS.

Both expand rather than mediate the experience of AIDS, and do so with precision rather than frenzy, at the very same moment that *Rent* became an unprecedented smash success.

GAY MALE CONTENT AND THE THEATRICAL CONTEXT FOR <u>RENT</u>

In the 1995–96 season, plays by gay men with overtly gay content were plentiful. At that moment white gay male theater seemed to have become a normalized voice on the New York stage as long as it didn't have too much to say about homophobia. One outstanding exception was the March opening of *A Fair Country* by Jon Robin Baitz. In retrospect, I think that what really appealed to me was that he managed to put familial homophobia and its impact on a gay man's life front and center, giving it as much dramatic power as the other subjects: colonialism, apartheid, and white complicity. Baitz was able to achieve a very difficult and personally challenging balance between conveying the truth of his own experience of homophobia alongside the truth of his own experience of white supremacy. I have seen too many plays about how the white straight man is oppressed by the black or gay or female, and yet I have never seen a play by a heterosexual about how heterosexuals have manipulated and profited from homophobia. By articulating both sides of the divide of privilege and oppression, Baitz created a hugely important work.

The play is set in the 1970s, and the Burgess family is living in Durban, South Africa, because the father, Harry (Laurence Luckenbill), has a low-level diplomatic posting. His wife, Patrice (Judith Ivey), is trying to both adapt to and resist the role of white mistress in apartheid. As the play opens, she has just been in an abusive struggle with a Zulu maid named Edna, on whom she called the vile Durban police, an act that goes against the stated values of this

American family. Both she and her son Gil (Matt McGrath) are hysterical. They have become trapped by the dramatic racism of apartheid and increasingly resigned to the self-disgust of their complicity.

Their situation is revealed even further when the elder son, Alec (Dan Futterman), comes to visit from New York. Alec challenges Gil's increasing participation in the apartheid mentality. Gil, the squeaky and frightened gay son, rejects Alec's encouragement to transcend this role, for Gil's complicity with his situation is the only thing that makes him normal. So, when Alec offers the ultimate acceptance, to have Gil move in with him in New York and become part of his world, Gil has to make a choice between the family of his future (his brother) and the family of his past (his parents). Gil chooses the past with its illusion of safety that we, the adult audience, know will inevitably grow into stagnation. Gil must reject his brother's courage and love because Gil is so dependent on his parents' approval, he just doesn't have the guts for change.

The real evil heart of this family is not Patrice, the fall guy or the erratic, distressed, inappropriately angry mother. It is not Gil, the cowardly fag. It is not Alec, the devoted man of conscience. For, after all accounts of their flaws, the question remains, why are these three people wrapped in a system that is not their burden by birth? Why? Because this is Harry's job, and Harry's job is destroying his family. But the impossibility of anyone ever suggesting that he quit his job is the great silence and dramatic center of this play. Harry's position is unquestioned.

Patrice is destroyed by her loyalty to her husband, for it requires her to remain in a constant state of inadequacy. The sons, too, must also be kept inadequate so that no one can ever surpass the father. So kindly, so right, so worried about his "troubled" wife that his supremacy can't possibly be demonized, Harry is a nice guy. He is too "good" to be displaced, no matter what the cost to everyone else. His position is the source of rage, and everyone else must pay the price as Dad stays forever off the hook.

Usually, in a play of this nature, the "political" character is reduced to a useless, silly, impotent clown. But in *A Fair Country* the audience knows what has happened in South Africa. We know that this is one place on earth where the kinds of people usually denounced in bourgeois theater are actually acknowledged as having achieved a kind of justice. So, in this play, finally, the burden of evil falls on someone else besides the man of faith.

Realizing that Baitz brought off a hopeful resolution without watering down the truth was the perfect antidote to the defenses I'd been hearing about *Rent*. So many people claimed that the truth about A I D S wouldn't be entertaining, and that a good theatrical experience relied on falsity. But Baitz doesn't soften the message. He doesn't make it palatable. He makes it true, and he follows through. Suddenly the angry son is right to be angry, the bitter son is right to be bitter, the crazy mother is right to be crazy. So, when in the final scene fate alone has determined that Patrice and Gil will be free to have the relationship they always deserved, it is a happy ending.

There was another openly gay show of great significance to this discussion, by two out gay men that year. In many ways, it was an authentic product of everything *Rent* falsely claimed to stand for. It was *Hot Keys,* by Jeff Weiss and carlos ricardo martinez (a.k.a. Murphy), and it played at P S 122 every Friday and Saturday night at midnight throughout the spring of 1996.

I have been watching carlos and Jeffrey's work since 1980, and there is still nothing I can say here that will convey the experience of seeing it. It is hard to separate myth from reality with them, but vaguely the story goes that they met thirty-six years ago when Jeff was a young hustler. Carlos got him off the street and into theater, which saved his life. Their first piece, at the legendary Café Cino, was a coming-home party for a young man who had just returned from getting a lobotomy. Since then their work has taken on many incarnations. I first became aware of it when I saw carlos's plays *Teddy and the Social Worker* and the unforgettable *Art the Rat* at the Performing Garage. Carlos's style, at that time, was to treat every performance like a rehearsal and every rehearsal like a performance. So, it was not unusual to see him jump up on stage in the middle of the show and make the actors "take it back," do the scene one more time.

I then started to attend *That's How the Rent Gets Paid,* Jeff's long-running soap opera in the format now used by *Hot Keys,* using the best actors in town in the early eighties (Ron Vawter as Detective Persky, Mary Shultz as his wife, Nona, and Dorothy Cantwell as Izzy, my favorite lesbian character to ever grace the stage). He also had a cast of actors from his hometown, Allentown, Pennsylvania, who intermixed with the New Yorkers. Jeff presented a new three-to-six-hour installment every single week. It told the ongoing story of Connie Gearheart, an actor, and his vicious double, Bjorn, a Finnish serial killer. Both parts were played by Jeff. And of course, the classic moment in this extravaganza was when Connie and Bjorn actually met and fucked at the Saint Mark's Baths. It made no difference that both parts were played by the same actor. *That's How the Rent Gets Paid* brought Nikki Paraiso into the family mix. This musician, performance artist, actor, and singer is a mainstay of New York off-off. He has been their musical director ever since, and provides an illusion of sanity, calm, and a lovely charm, no matter how far out of hand the proceedings may get.

After that show, Jeff and carlos performed out of the Acting Academy, a storefront underneath their apartments on East Tenth Street. This was in the middle of the violent gentrification of the East Village and carlos's plays served as a real people's theater of outrage against the destruction of the neighborhood. Songs like "Dear Mister Mayor" from *Teddy* were on-stage manifestations of increasingly public protests. His hand-painted signs on walls and dumpsters were visible daily reminders of opposition to the occupation of the neighborhood by mounted police, the influx of cocaine culture through the art galleries, and the removal of Latinos from the neighborhood. Going to shows at the Academy was a real treat. A number of times I showed up with a friend, to find that we were the only people in the audience. That didn't stop the cast from doing all three hours. Then, afterward, Jeff and carlos would serve wine and good bread, cheese with delicious honey mustard. They never created a separation between themselves and the audience. They never put themselves above the audience or the neighborhood.

But the neighborhood was disappearing, nonetheless. Jeff and carlos have always resisted the phoniness of the art world, and they responded to East Village hype in a similar vein by not advertising their shows, not inviting the press, and not applying for grants. Jeff did do some work in the early performance spaces. I remember seeing him and Dorothy Cantwell at the 8BC Club. The audience members knew to bring signature flashlights, and those two would reenact scenes from *That's How the Rent Gets Paid* under the eerie glow.

Flashlights were part of carlos's theatrical method. Even today, he is always in the light booth making flickering choices, emphasizing and then undercutting the action with unpredictable illumination. His method also called for Jeff's line-up of diverse characters to be distinguished only by slight changes of clothing. A new hat, a different jacket, rolled-up sleeves. Everything that happened on stage could be conveyed emotionally; it didn't have to be expensive.

But time was passing. Jeff had long had a reputation as "the greatest actor in New York City," but he chose not to work professionally because of his commitment to his and carlos's own vision of theater. Finally, somewhere around his fiftieth birthday, Jeff took the plunge. The story is that Kevin Kline slipped a note under Jeff's front door asking him to play the ghost opposite Kline's *Hamlet* at the Public Theater, known to Jeff's friends as "The Pubic." (Jeff and carlos have never had a telephone. If you stand on the corner of First Avenue and Tenth Street you can see Jeff making business calls on the pay phone surrounded by the drug dealers who work that spot.)

59

The ensuing performance was so spectacular that it moved Frank Rich, then chief theater critic at the *Times,* to comment that this was the first time in the history of *Hamlet* that the Prince's relationship with the ghost was stronger than his relationship with Ophelia. This was followed by a string of commercial roles in such plays as *Mastergate* on Broadway, *Our Town* at Lincoln Center, *The Play's the Thing* at the Roundabout, and more work at the Public. Jeff was at the glowing center of every review, but carlos made sure it did not go to his head.

In 1991 they decided to return to the stage with another long-running soap opera, *Hot Keys.* The title refers to an image Jeff had that all the gay men who had gone through the bathhouses had the outline of their locker key burned onto their wrists by the steam and that this was the sign of who could be carrying the dreaded "Taint." The first production was an odd mix of yuppie actors from the Naked Angels Company that Jeff had met while working commercially and his old downtown independent stalwarts. Kristin Johnson, a member of the Atlantic Theater Company, who was brilliant as the original Vicki Scheiskopf in *Hot Keys* now plays an alien on the hit T V show *Third Rock from the Sun.* But the downtowners are still below Fourteenth Street and will stay there as long as rent control lasts. And they were the center of the 1996 production at PS 122.

Still, none of this background information can convey the love and generosity at the core of the *Hot Keys* experience. A community of bonded, die-hard fans are as essential to the craziness and joy of the show as the actors themselves. The audience lines up, waiting to get into the theater and carefully reads the program for that evening's show to see which actors are playing which parts, which favorite scenes are being tried out again, which charcters are appearing for the first time. We all join in together to sing "the traditional opening number," or wait to see, each week, which member of the Glee Club is going to sing carlos's signature song, "Please Let Love Pass Me By."

As Jeff once explained to me in reference to the AIDS crisis: "However sad and sorrowful our losses, the *fact* of daily life (read *performance*) should go on. This is how Murphy feels and I agree with him as ever. We have a moral and ethical obligation to persist in the living of real (as opposed to 'reel') time. That is the power of theater. We're all in this together, at the *same* time. We're totally engaged in being human together, sharing the identical instants as our time advances, parallel, in unison."

It's so bizarre to have to compare this vision of what it is to be an artist with the depiction of artists in *Rent*. I never knew Jonathan Larson, but the strange myth that has emerged out of the problems he caused me makes me actually feel sorry for him, because he missed out on wonderful experience. At first I thought that Larson's rejection of this generosity of spirit was rooted in some imperial yuppiedom that colonized everything that was in its path. But as I looked more closely, I now think the truth is even sadder than that. The falseness of his depiction of what it is to be an artist went against even the truth of his own life. In *Rent,* Mark, the straight white male protagonist of *Rent* is a video artist. His dilemma, believe it or not, is that MTV is calling him, hounding him to "sell out," and he can't decide whether or not he wants to. This premise, alone, is so preposterous as to be nauseating. It has nothing to do with what artists really experience, especially East Village artists of the era Larson is caricaturing. The fact of Larson himself dying of an aortic aneurism, after twice receiving incompetent care in an emergency room, makes the distortion even more pathological. In other words, he died because he was poor.

I don't know much about him, but I do know that he was working as a waiter at the time of *Rent*. Having been a waitress myself for ten years, I know that that is not a sign of comfort. He was poor because he was an artist. If he had the money, he would have gone to a private doctor. But he didn't, and so he died. Yet his depiction of the life of an artist is one of spoiled suburbanites who have nothing better to do and who choose their deprivations. I am sure that Larson was a composer because he had to be. It was a compulsion inside him that could not be stifled. Given the punishing atmosphere for artists in our society, there is really no other viable explanation. But he lied about it to please an audience, and then he died of it. If he had been exposed to (which he may have been) Jeff's vision of a community of artists and audience united under "moral and ethical" questions, and, more importantly, open to it, *Rent* would have been quite a different production and not just a product.

At the same time that gay men were making work with gay male protagonists on the New York stage, there were significant revivals of two of Tennessee Williams's plays during Don's and my tenure at the *New York Press.* Both are relevant to our discussion, one in terms of gay male content and one in terms of lesbian content. Despite the enforced coding of his day, both of Williams's plays provoked me to do a lot of thinking about gay issues on stage.

Suddenly Last Summer was produced at Circle in the Square Uptown in October 1995. It was an uninspired production with a strangely unfocused performance by Elizabeth Ashley, but the play was resonating faster than the speed of light. It transcended the museum in which it had been encased and illuminated our own time.

The play concerns Sebastian Venable, a closeted gay man who dies brutally before the piece begins. His cousin, Catherine, is the only witness to the truth of his life, a story that no one in the family wants to hear.

This may not be the traditional plot summary of *Suddenly Last Summer,* but it doesn't take long for the modern urgencies of the play to become clear. This is a work that really allows us to look at the complex position of women who survive gay men. After all, Nan Goldin's infamous show at Artists' Space (which was the first art event to be targeted by Jesse Helms's then-new campaign against arts funding) called us *Witnesses* to their vanishing.

Sebastian's mother, Violet Venable, will do anything to keep Catherine from telling the truth about her son. She doesn't want to know that he was a homosexual. She doesn't want to know what the impact of her own homophobia was on his life. Like all homophobes, she wants to pretend that her vulgar evisceration of him was morally good and pure. That his homosexuality was simultaneously non-existent and pathological.

Continuing the historic conspiracy between families and psychiatry to punish sexuality, Violet manages to get Catherine locked up in the local nuthouse. But that hasn't killed the girl's insistence on the facts. Violet then engages Dr. Sugar, a friendly psychiatrist with a sinister agenda, to interview Catherine at the Venable estate. The agreement is that if he incarcerates her in an even more severe institution, Catherine's future lobotomy will earn a large donation for Dr. Sugar's research.

Catherine is more than the girl who gets punished for telling the truth. She is not just an empty receptacle of Sebastian's life. She also has her own life. She is an aware, rebellious woman who followed an erotic and imaginative path far outside the acceptable boundaries of her family and gender. It was her awareness of her own desires, her strong oppositional insistence on self, that led her to a friendship with Sebastian in the first place. Her punishment is predicated, not only on what she knows about Sebastian, but also on what she knows about her own female existence. For this, too, she must be destroyed.

Here we get to an even more complex subject, which can also be easily excavated from Williams's play: the dialogic relationship between women and gay men. Like many fag hags and lesbians who pal around with gay men, Catherine had a relationship with Sebastian of mutual appreciation and mutual use. She used him for safety. He was the only man she could be with who would allow her to move freely through the world. He made it possible for her to have love affairs, make scenes, travel abroad, and still have male protection.

For Sebastian, Catherine was his measure of truth. She knew who he really was and loved him because of it. He also used her both as a beard, an illusion of heterosexuality to smooth his path, and at the same time he used her free sexuality to (in the most famous line of the play) "procure." That is, he used her to attract young men whom he then would seduce or buy off for sex. So, when he died, she not only lost him, she lost her safeguard in a world hostile to oppositional women. This is a protection available only at a cost, true, but a lower cost than marriage.

The racial issues at the core of *Suddenly Last Summer* also cannot be ignored. Sebastian took Catherine to Mexico where he bought sex from the starving dark young boys who end up murdering him. One day, when he was "as white as the weather," Catherine tells Dr. Sugar, these hungry boys came up to the restaurant where the two cousins were seated and started yelling for bread. "They made gobbling noises with their little black mouths, stuffing their little black fists with frightful grins." Deprived of his personhood within his own culture, Sebastian relied on his only area of supremacy to create a theater for his homosexuality. And the people he exploited ultimately got their revenge. This play resonates very strongly with Baitz's *A Fair Country,* in its relationship between familial homophobia and white supremacy.

When I was watching the play I remember feeling that the flat retelling that emphasizes the "unspoken secret" is a tired and safe interpretation. But to get under the skin of *Suddenly Last Summer* requires a production that is more inventive and far more courageous.

THE LESBIAN THEATRICAL CONTEXT OF RENT

One of the frustrations provoked by the really nasty depiction of lesbian love in *Rent* was that lesbian writers with lesbian content are so excluded from the city's mainstages. That the lesbian lovers in *Rent* do little besides bicker would be immaterial if this was but one of a hundred different available depictions. But when *Rent* is the only visible rendition of lesbian life on the Broadway stage, that's an entirely different matter. It is one thing to misrepresent a group of people when they have a voice within hearing distance. But the misrepresentation of lesbians on the New York stage is taking place in a void of response. There is a long, rich tradition of lesbians in stand-up comedy and solo performance from Moms Mabley to Betsy Damon to Danitra Vance. But it is a different story when you look at the lonely, fragile history of lesbian *playwriting* here in New York.

It is hard to find primary lesbian content on stage by an uncloseted writer before *Fefu and Her Friends* by Maria Irene Fornes in 1977. Or maybe it was Corinne Jacker's *Harry Outside* at the Circle Repertory Company in 1975. But, although each was sealed with a passionate kiss, both of these plays contained their lesbian content in subplots. Lesbian content was primary on stage at Medusa's Revenge at 10 Bleecker Street, the first theater in the world willing to produce our work. It was founded by Ana Maria Simo and others whose names I do not know, in New York City, in the early seventies. Now Medusa's Revenge has never made it into any of the official histories of feminist or lesbian theater but it lasted for about ten years and was run by Ana and her lover Migali, an actress who worked with Tom Eyen, the notorious gay playwright who died of AIDS. Both women were Cuban refugees.

Ana has been an out lesbian writing plays with overt content for over twenty years. I have for more than fifteen. Ira Jeffries, Holly Hughes, and a number of others have as well, including Joan Schenkar (although she calls herself a sapphist) and Susan Miller. But the number of openly lesbian playwrights with consistently open lesbian content who have been able to keep going over the years is quite small. Most writers daring to try were driven out, and after two or three productions either quit playwriting or produced work with repressed, secondary, or coded lesbian characters. Theater is a very expensive hobby. It is enormously punishing to be playwright of any stripe. But lesbian playwrights have faced a special history of isolation and obstruction.

In the early eighties, a handful of us doing this work were forced together even though we had nothing in common. We had different aesthetic sensibilities, different ethical values, and different degrees of talent. The only thing we shared was a common exclusion from the rest of the theatrical world because we were out in our work.

In some ways it is a reward for our determination that in the last few years we've seen established writers becoming more willing to queer their pitch at the same time that a new generation of younger people are staring out, "out." So in addition to Miller, Jeffries, Simo, et al., it is now possible to see openly lesbian work on stage by Paula Vogel, Tina Landau, Phyllis Nagy, Claire Chafee, Shay Youngblood, Anne Harris, Emma Donohue, Kate Ryan, Honour Molloy, and many, many others. But, in the historical long view, lesbian playwriting is filled with small output, frustrated efforts, and the startling but still dominant fact that even today the most prominent lesbian playwrights are closeted.

In the late seventies and early eighties, a heyday for grassroots organizations created by women artists, even the so-called avant garde performance spaces like PS 122 and the Kitchen were not programming this work. As far as press coverage went, the daily papers ignored us, so our only possibilities of exposure were in sporadic coverage by a profoundly sexist gay press, occasional interest from short-lived progressive papers, a women's press that did not understand art, or the *Village Voice.* It is not evident whether, in the long run, the *Voice* did us more harm than good. After the departure of jill johnston, lesbian critics at the *Voice* were often closeted and therefore, by definition ill equipped to evaluate this boldly out and evolving theatrical movement.

The press is a complex obstacle, because public discourse with critics and journalists is a real David-and-Goliath venture with the twist being that David usually loses. If you stand up to them, you get punished. People who make theater on waitress tips have no way of responding to the power of corporate newspapers. But, if you want to be Zen about it, the long-term price is a lot higher when artists do not attempt to open dialogue with the people controlling their ability to earn a living and make work. Frankly, a personal vendetta by Jesse Helms has not shown to be as devastating to an artist's development and career as a personal vendetta by a writer at the *Village Voice*. That's why I find a lot of the "anti-censorship" rhetoric to be really hypocritical when it is propelled by critics with territorial monopolies.

When the *Voice* finally did start to review our work in the early eighties, it was in a contained way, in that we would only be compared to one another. Typically, the critic would comment on three different pieces of lesbian work and say why Holly was better than Carmelita or why Reno was better than Holly. We were never positioned as part of the larger theatrical culture. Ironically, as the critics systematically contained us, the critics themselves were systematically contained, in that we were rarely reviewed by anyone other than a lesbian. This underlined our marginality and reinforced in everyone's mind that we were not important and no one besides other freaks had any reason to pay attention to our work. The result of this kind of containment was brutal on our psyches, because our closest friends and greatest supporters became our worst competitors. And, most important, we had no understanding of how entrenched the obstacles against us really were. We could not see why no degree of merit or effort could shake them while the men and straight friends among us seemed to move ever forward.

As our audiences grew, it became clear that marginal established theaters that had once excluded us, like PS 122 et al., would soon have to let us in. But in the spirit of the *Village Voice*'s militant tokenism, only one of us, or one clique, or one aesthetic sensibility could have any credibility. In fact, this unspoken quota system is still present in many places where one lesbian play will be produced or reviewed or one out lesbian grant application will be awarded, regardless of how many women's work was of merit. This is particularly painful when you realize that many of us have virtually nothing in common aesthetically except our integrity about our homosexuality, and yet we are all made to compete for the same slots.

At any rate, the few out lesbian critics quickly became factionalized and identified with particular artists. This, of course, is a rampant problem of critics. In order to have credibility, critics must be associated with artists who become successful. So, often the same critic will vote for the person to receive an award for the work they gave a good review to, in order to back up the grant. This mutual professional dependency in a world as small as lesbian playwriting means that any new individual or aesthetic or any oppositional expression becomes a threat to the professional status of the critic, who is already identified with a particular artist. The critic, of course, gets *paid* for her work, unlike the artist, who loses money. With tokenism this rigidly enforced, thank God the gay men at the *New York Times* started, around 1990, to review lesbian work. Ironically, although they are less comprehending of lesbian cultural reference, they are often more supportive, ecumenical, and open minded, since their own reputations and futures as critics are not wrapped up in which lesbian sensibilities receive public exposure. The men have credibility beyond their subject while the lesbian critics often do not. Straight people are not in this picture at all. While some straight male critics have supported gay male work, there is no straight man out there championing lesbian theater.

But the problem with being dependent on gay male critics or terrifically encouraging straight women like Laurie Stone at the *Voice* to get fair coverage for new developments in lesbian theater is that they cannot serve as the kind of personal network of mentors behind the scenes for us that men will for other men. As lesbian playwrights, when we each undertook to pioneer this endeavor we dreamed of a criticism that would encourage, support, and invigorate our work. There are no out lesbians reviewing theater in the daily press. Thus, we cannot build the networks of power and support or make the connections upon which viable careers depend, because there are so few people with power to connect with. There is no one to mentor us. Straight people don't see us as equals, gay men are increasingly better but still unwilling to extend material support our way and share resources on an equal basis, and the closet cases are still racing off in the other direction.

Another important factor in the historic repression of lesbian work, interestingly, was lack of academic credentials. I can't recall a single playwright from that time who had an MFA. We did not come from Yale and NYU and Brown. This work was entirely community-based. We did not take classes in performance studies. We went to shows, usually at the very theaters who discriminated against us, something I still do regularly. We admired closeted lesbian artists and read newspapers that ghettoized and humiliated us. We were completely devoid of institutional support. There was only one entity that loved us: the audience. I have always appreciated and derived great pleasure from grassroots audiences, with their wide diversity of arts backgrounds. The performers were from mixed-class backgrounds, and so were the audiences. There were no high ticket prices and no tuition bills.

It was a difficult but fascinating conundrum, for while we got no reviews, no grants, no workshops, no staged readings, and no dramaturgy and had to produce our own shows, we had the one thing that institutional playwrights lacked, a passionate audience. It has always amazed me how much the audiences loved and appreciated precommodification gay and lesbian work. It is actually shocking to go to a dominant-culture theater and see the dominant-culture playwright's audiences, who are supremely disengaged from the work. However, as satisfying as it has been to have audiences that consistently love and need the play, the discrepancy between the urgency of that relationship and the complete lack of social support or acknowledgment is personally very hard to take. The more the marginalized audience loves it, the clearer it becomes for the playwright to what extent she is being professionally punished for the lesbian content of her work. And ultimately this base in the community and lack of university connections has been an overwhelming factor in our continued isolation from structures of support. In many ways, because we were out, we were institutionally underdeveloped.

After all, one of the great ironies of history is that the people who make change are not the ones who benefit from it. As those with enough integrity to be out made the world safe for homosexuality, the world produced its own version of homosexuality and kept the originators out. So that now, those of us who developed a grassroots audience and made it impossible for the world to deny the existence of homosexuality, now have our audience taken away by mainstream facsimile product. Instead of our work taking its deserved place in the broad spectrum of recognized American cultural life, the actual is supplanted by the distorted imitation.

Theater has its particular problems in this area. Of all the art worlds I've worked in, theater is by far the most restricted. The exclusion of work by women in general is strictly maintained. It has been amazing to watch theater emerge as a force for cultural reaction, and I don't just mean *CATS*. There has surfaced, recently, what I think of as the Theater of Resentment. It is most notably represented by works like Mamet's *Oleanna,* but has increasingly become standard fare in emerging work by younger white straight males. The formula is as follows: the white straight male protagonist encounters some exoticized Other; women, Blacks, Latinos, gays or some combination thereof. This Other then proceeds to be the catalyst for the protagonist's catharsis by manipulating her or his disenfranchised status in a sneaky and untruthful way. By the end, both the superiority and the centrality of the protagonist is reaffirmed be-

70

cause he has had an emotional transformation through his encounter with this Other and is now even better than he was before.

What is most insidious about this pervasive school of work is that it maintains a liberal veneer by simply including outsider characters in the world of the play, which then stands in stark contrast to their invisibility historically. *Rent* acknowledges that lesbians exist; therefore it claims to be tolerant. The fact that it repeatedly inscribes lesbian relationships as unstable, bickering, and emotionally pathological is the required conceit. For, in the end, white makes right. It is a theater rooted in the idea that people who believed they were superior and should naturally dominate are now being told that their position is simply an accident of birth. They desperately want to contain and neutralize any effort to make them acknowledge the construction of their dominance. So, they create caricatures of us and confine us within the prison of their plays. It is what Marcuse called "repressive tolerance." It was with this history and this understanding, that I stepped into my role as theater critic, observer on a field of bounty in which my kind was not allowed to participate.

Don and I saw two significant works by openly lesbian writers with primary lesbian content in the '95–'96 season. Given the inability of out writers to get full productions for multicharacter plays with lesbian protagonists, both were solo performance pieces. In February 1996 we attended a performance of Susan Miller's *My Left Breast* at the Ohio Theater. This was a revival of the earlier Obie-winning show. The evening we went was, coincidentally, a benefit for the American Cancer Society. The audience was 90 percent female, ages twenty to sixty, coats ranging from second-hand cloth to full-length mink. For years I have been watching plays about A I D S while sitting in rooms full of people with A I D S, but this is the first play I've ever seen about a woman with cancer in a room of women with cancer. As A I D S has become increasingly unpalatable as a subject for gay art, gay men have increasingly been moving to

71

other diseases. Women with diseases have become metaphors for men. In Susan Miller's show, women are women and cancer is cancer. So there were only a handful of men in the room that evening.

The audience members greeted each other with formal familiarity. They introduced their friends to the other insiders. "This is Edith," one said. "She's my support system."

Then Miller comes on stage. She looks like an older Ellen DeGeneres: sharp nose, blue eyes, boyish hair, brown saddle shoes. "I miss it," she says. "But it's not my mind. It's not the roof over my head. . . . It's not my courage or my faith."

First, she tells us that she's wearing a prosthesis. Then she comes out as a lesbian. The audience was unusually quiet. Like her, they have cancer. They can't abandon her now for being queer. Not in the first five minutes of the show. Besides, Miller is a real writer. The real thing. As the piece soars, we luxuriate in every telling detail of this crackerjack writer's conversational poetry, her casual philosophy, and loving truths. As she tells us the story of her life, the mundane details of everyday concerns captivate. The sound of an ex-lover's name resounds as universally as moonlight.

"This is my body where the past and the future collide. All at once, timely."

And that ex-lover, Franny, is even more important to the story than the cancer. Because Miller's ability to love and be loved is more of who she is than her disease.

I look around at the audience. A perfect blond in a perfect suit with pink nails and high heels is listening intently, responding, laughing out loud, her legs crossed, and arms clutched around her middle. Two older Jewish women overtly sulk, ensuring by their insistently raised eyebrows that everyone else in the theater knows they don't approve. Just because they have cancer doesn't mean they have to associate with that other stuff. Things are breaking down.

Now Miller is talking about her son. She's sending him to day camp, to Brandeis, telling him about her cancer, ironing his shirt.

Can she win over the judging Jewish ladies with motherhood? They start unwrapping candy, the kind encased in layers of cellophane. "The Crinklers," the late George Osterman used to call them. I guess they were feeling something.

"I didn't lose my hair—I lost my period," she says from the stage.

Hot flashes. Big laugh. They're with her now. Menopause theater. But, oh-oh, there's Franny again. Being left by Franny is as great a loss as the breast in question. But Franny's departure is static, an obsession. The cancer has a longer narrative arc. Fractured ribs. Bone loss. "Is the structure of everything dissolving?" Tumor search. Doctors, doctors, doctors.

When she talks about doctors, the audience comes around. Nods of understanding, laughter of the informed, grunts of the insider. There is only one stern-faced refusenik in the front row who has managed to fall asleep. Yes. No. Yes. No.

"Your doctor says *positive.* Your lover says *it's over.* . . . And you say good-bye to the person you thought you were. . . . I'm going to show you my scar in a minute."

Do they really want to see it? I wonder, trying to catch the audience vibe as we wait in anticipation. *Will she really do that?* And, what about me? *What do I feel?* And suddenly it occurs to me that I am a participant here, not an observer. I feel that this is my future. I feel that the presence of cancer in my life is inevitable. It is there now and it will always be there. Me, or if not me, so many that I know. That's why I'm involved with the audience's judgment. That woman up there might be my future.

"We are still sexy," she is saying. "We are still here." Then the lights dim, she opens her shirt and shows her scar. But she's already given us so much of herself that the stigma is gone. It's just another part of her life. This play made me laugh, but it did not make me cry. I leave the theater thinking that it all turned out okay. *That scar is something I can live with,* I realize, transformed from having watched her work. And I remember that this is something I have never felt when watching a film or a play or reading a book or hearing a song where the woman with a disease is only a metaphor for an unacceptable man.

The following month we went to the Public Theater. In my life as an artist, the Public has never produced a full play by an out lesbian with primary lesbian content. They did do a work by Susan Miller in 1978, but I was still a teenager. The exclusion of lesbian work by the Public is a long story. My early collaborator Robin Epstein called it Joe Papp's Private Theater. But recently they have been allowing lesbian solo acts with limited runs. And so, until they crack the glass ceiling and let us into play production, one-woman shows are all we will get. Fortunately this one was by Marga Gomez, so the pleasure was guaranteed.

The sidewalk in front of the Second Avenue Deli is lined with stars. You can find Boris Tomashefsky, Miriam Kressyn, and Ida Kaminska's names engraved in the cement. As a child I saw an old Miriam Kressyn in *Yoshe Kalb* at the Maurice Schwartz Yiddishe Arts Theater. *She was so beautiful,* my grandmother sighed, thinking of herself. Later, I was a stagehand in the same theater for the memorial tribute to Charles Ludlum. Now it is a multiplex with ornate Jewish stars carved into the ceilings. There were actors on the Yiddish stage that were as talented, as beloved, and as committed as any Hollywood star. There are singers in the Chinese opera that surpass the most famous M T V bimbo. There are gay icons with devoted followings that no straight person can name.

Marga Gomez's show, *A Line around the Block,* honored her father, Willy Chevalier, a Cuban vaudevillian who played Latin *teatros* in New York City. Gomez was born in a trunk, and this clear-eyed tribute to her father is also an investigation of how she, too, became a performer. But there is even a more poignant layer of identification in this piece, because Gomez is also a seasoned veteran of the gay circuit. She knows from years of personal experience what the world of marginalized show biz is all about. Whether

74

it is Harlem in the sixties or San Francisco in the eighties, the atmosphere of cheesy clubs, low wages, underground stardom, and its accompanying humiliations are very much the same.

Gomez is drop-dead gorgeous and very funny. But it is her boyish awkwardness and open heart that has always made her so compelling on stage. Plus she's had the integrity of being out of the closet, bringing her whole self to her work, and this piece is no exception. The story of her father's never-ending enthusiasm for doomed schemes and love of theater is intercut with little Marga's first serious crush—in this case, on Latin diva Irma Pagan, who appears in one of her father's variety nights.

Like Anna Deveare Smith, Gomez plays men as her neutral self. Her father, with his ever-present cup of coffee, never stops making plans to simultaneously depose Castro, open another show, and impress his ex-wife. Every step of his decline is explained as something special, something wonderful. "I could wash the windows," he tells his daughter. "But this way the *publico* could not look in." Or promising to become a great success and build a swimming pool in the backyard of his one-room apartment. But Gomez does not judge him too harshly, for she knows how much delusion is required to keep going in the theater.

Gomez plays all the roles without pretension. This is far from those anguished multicharacter actor things. The show is funny, touching, and very original. Her characters run the gamut of old Latino New York, a dramatically underrepresented part of what Ann Douglas has coined "Mongrel Manhattan." By the end of the show, we know everyone in the neighborhood. A nosy Dominican bodega owner treats every purchase of Cafe Bustelo as an opportunity for a full interrogation on Gomez's family news. Willy puts on live advertisements for Cafe Pico between acts, and Marga's mother plays a vamp to her father's *Vampiro*. But the star turn is Gomez's rendition of the beloved Pagan as something somewhere between Ann Margaret and Barry White.

In one scene, Gomez recounts the favored stars of the *teatros*. She goes through a number of performers, all of whose names are unknown to the non-Latinos in the audience. Then she comes to one particular performer. "She was bigger than Elvis," Gomez assures us. "Audiences loved her." And we know what she means. When your life is never on stage, and Willy Chevalier or Marga Gomez have the guts, the drive, the courage, the delusion, and the endless enthusiasm necessary to get the show up there, they are heroes. Appropriation, no matter how appealing, can never be as powerful to those being appropriated as the real thing. And there are certainly people who will come out of this show transformed and gratified in a way that they never could get from Elvis. I'm one of them.

One of the most interesting lesbian subtext experiences that season emerged in a revival of Tennessee Williams's *The Night of the Iguana* at the Roundabout in April with Cherry Jones, the toast of Broadway, in the lead role of Hannah Wilkes, the spinster from Nantucket. The casting of Jones, a superior actor and an out lesbian, allowed new levels of resonance to Williams's play. Long a fan, I had already seen Jones on Broadway in her Tony-award–winning role in *The Heiress.* On opening night of *The Heiress,* her Catherine Sloper, an awkward, wealthy nineteenth-century New Yorker, was being wooed by one Morris Townsend, a possible gigolo. When Morris gave her her first kiss, Jones's passion on stage was so complete and real it was almost too intimate to observe. It was the kind of expression of passion that I have personally only seen one-on-one and never so convincingly on stage. That night, by the end of the play, Sloper soberly vowed to live the rest of her life without men, and I was left with a curious emotion. Where was the bitter old maid that we'd all expected? Instead, Jones offered us a woman whose entire life had just begun, filled with possibility.

Five months later, on a hot July Wednesday night after all the rave reviews and awards, I went to see *The Heiress* again. This time the kiss meant very little. She was pleased, ecstatic within the limits of her emotional life, but the white hot core of desire was not there. The kiss was now all about other matters, supremely the possibility of being loved by another person, of existing outside of the realm of her father's power. Consequently, the ending was also different. By this point, Catherine Sloper's understanding of what her future could and would be was so informed that the knowledge had driven her mad. She was wild, completely out of control. That is when the passion emerged. The two different renditions added up to a very subversive performance. And everyone in New York theater seemed to know how brilliant it was, but few were able to articulate why.

So I went to the Roundabout's revival of *Iguana* with great expectations. My expectations were met, but not in any way that I had predicted or imagined. And it left questions that have kept me reeling ever since.

The play is set in Mexico in 1940 at the broken-down tourist compound run by Maxine (Marsha Mason). She's being visited by Shannon (William Peterson), an alcoholic former minister who was locked out of his church for fornication and heresy. He now leads guided tours through Mexico for lady teachers from Texas. Shannon is having his latest nervous breakdown, compounded by yet another one-night stand with yet another underaged girl. Enter Hannah Jelkes and her grandfather Nonno (Lawrence McCauley), who have traveled together for twenty-five years working the tourist trade with their sketches and poetic recitations. They're broke, and she desperately needs to hustle everyone in sight from Maxine, to four ultra-vixen Nazi tourists, to the busload of angry Texas schoolmarms. *Iguana* is a tough play for a 1990s audience. Its beauty lies in the relationships between the characters, but there is a lot of business and many hurdles to leap before you get to those transcendent moments.

There are two crucial relationships at the center of Fall's production—Hannah and Shannon, and Hannah and Maxine. Mason plays Maxine as a down-to-earth middle-aged woman who won't give up pleasure but is still wise enough to know what real friendship is. She values other people, and even though she sometimes has to bully them into letting her get close to them, she's willing to be the fall guy because she knows that in the end, everyone will be better off.

What was new and fascinating in this production is what was going on between the women. Maxine is a type we all know. She likes men, wants Shannon either in her bed or in her world, and she will fight all comers for her guy. She thinks she knows Hannah's type, the repressed Puritan who, despite airs, is going to fight tooth and nail for the same guy. The surprise here is that Maxine really *doesn't* know Hannah, and neither do we. There is compassion and empathy between Hannah and Shannon, but not romance. Yet Maxine can't see this. So the scenes between the two women are revealingly lopsided. Maxine knows nothing about the kind of woman she's dealing with but she thinks she knows everything. Hannah really does know Maxine and plays all her cards with great care and strategic precision. Both women, being older and very self aware, attack and back off, threaten and give in by formula, not by explosive emotion. It is an oddly effective portrait of how fully formed women interact on a playing field where one is known and the other, obscure.

As for the Hannah/Shannon relationship, after having seen each other in various intimate states of degradation, Shannon finally pops the big question. Has Hannah ever known *love,* by which he means *sex.*

What follows is a story that is perverse on every level. You'll have to read the play to find out what it is. But what's important here is just that in Jones's performance, revealing her secret makes her no more vulnerable. While Hannah, as a woman of her temperament and position, must be very defended in order to survive, there has to be a place where the price is revealed. Her torment and resolve are simultaneously present, and her sexuality is present but under wraps—and she doesn't let anyone shake it up. If Shannon or Maxine could shake it up, even for a moment, if only we could see the crack, whether it is resentment or anger or deep desire (known or unknown), the performance would have resonated with even more strength.

On the other hand, I can defend Jones's performance as is, with equal enthusiasm. Of course, Hannah leaves the encounter with these two characters unchanged (except for the plot point death of her grandfather). Shannon and Maxine are not the kind of people who can deeply touch her. They are used to having power over people, but they do not have power over her. Their lack of ability to reach her shatters the age-old stereotype of the cold spinster. It is not Hannah who is deficient; it is Shannon. She has the capacity for love, but he is not enough for her to love. This interpretation shifts the traditional burden of deviance from the old maid to the handsome, tormented man—not an easy trick, since it goes against an entire culture's insistent baggage. And it takes an actor as disciplined and intelligent as Jones to be able to pull this off.

I don't know which option is more meaningful, and so I will just have to trust Jones. But the one place we can all agree that Falls and Jones are absolutely on target is when, despite all the advantageous circumstances surrounding Shannon's invitation to heterosexuality, Hannah never considers it for a moment. She doesn't back away; she's never coy. She just folds her arms and says no. We don't know how she would respond to an invitation to homosexuality, though, because Hannah's spinsterhood has a great deal to do with a refusal of gender conformity. When Shannon suggests that he and Hannah will "travel together," she responds with immediate and sarcastic refusal. When Jones answers, "I think the impracticality of the idea will appear much clearer to you in the morning," her subtext is screaming. She knows what she would have to give up.

Watching Jones work is not about watching perfection. It is about seeing human failings and vulnerabilities at the highest form of conscious articulation. And this production of *Iguana* again raised the need for a dramatic reinterpretation of Williams's work. Even with the taboos on homosexuality shifting to more complex terrain, the two Williams revivals in '95–'96 were both reticent. I remember an electric Super-8 film by the late Mark Morrisroe of Williams's *Hello from Bertha* with two drag queens. It would be great to let these plays breathe instead of staying mired in a desire to keep his characters' darkest secrets safely under wraps.

Ironically, this interpretation of *Iguana* cost me my job. Three days after it was published, the *New York Press* guys called Don and told him that we were fired. They didn't give a reason and had never expressed any displeasure. Don told them that they had to call me, too, and fire me to my face, but they never did. I guess that just treated us the way they would treat a straight couple. Since they never told me explicitly why this particular take was grounds enough for firing, I had to guess. I assume they decided, although did not consciously articulate, that lesbian subjectivity had no place in their newspaper. But I still believe that what I have to say about Cherry Jones's interpretation of Tennessee Williams is as legitimate a part of the cultural discourse as the dominant parameter. It is not special-interest, secondary, or marginal. It is part of American life and has a place within its most public discussions. This disapproving message, that we should contain ideas into a more "appropriate" place like the gay press, is a tedious threat that hangs over the professional lives of those of us who don't want to pathologize our own reality. But it is not worth capitulating to.

THE THEATRICAL CONTEXT OF BLACK WOMEN AND RENT

Race is a primary theme of *Rent*. It is simultaneously omnipresent and ignored. There are three casually interracial relationships, which also cross class. They are lesbian, gay, and heterosexual. But in all cases the race of the characters and particular mix of class, race, and sexuality is only decorative. The black middle-class lesbian has no difference of perspective or reality than the white heterosexual male or the Puerto Rican H I V-infected homeless, gay man. They are not acknowledged to have specificity of experience. Their lives do not influence their points of views, dreams, desires, ways of understanding, memories, predictions, prophesies, or patterns of logic. Nothing about the black lesbian character reflects or is a product of or is even influenced by her blackness. This level of distortion is central to the play's appeal because one of the most successful marketing falsities at the root of *Rent* is that "we" are all the same, as long as "we" are represented from a dominant cultural point of view.

The day that I am writing this chapter, the Sunday *New York Times* came out with two reviews of books with lesbian content. Openly gay Jeannette Winterson's *Gut Symmetries* was reviewed by a gay man with no literary background who is known primarily for being a fiscal conservative. Clearly the *Times* assigned him to the novel because they saw its lesbian content as automatically excluding the book from being treated like literature. Decidedly heterosexual Stewart O'Nan's novel, *The Speed Queen,* which features a lesbian protagonist, was reviewed by a prestigious heterosexual literary critic. The authentic expression was kept in its marginal place while the dominant cultural depiction of the same material is normatively positioned. Whose career benefits more from lesbian content, the lesbian novelist or the heterosexual male? In the theatrical context of *Rent* we see that Jonathan Larson's depiction of a black woman is for more commodifiable product than a black woman's depiction of herself.

There were a number of plays by black women that opened the same year as *Rent* that really stood out for me. I think they are worth remembering and looking at in some depth. In July of 1995 there was a revival of Ntozake Shange's *for colored girls who have considered suicide when the rainbow was enuf* at the New Federal

Theater. This black-directed theater is connected with the Henry Street Settlement House on the Lower East Side and has been run for years on a shoestring by Woodie King Jr. It is a community-based venue, and the audience comes from a wide range of theatrical experiences, so that there is a lot of talking back to the play and screaming out advice to characters. The audience really cares about what is happening on stage.

It was the twentieth anniversary production of this play, and the first thing I thought of, sitting in the audience, was Lorraine Hansberry. Shange's play sits curiously in the middle of the history of black gay and lesbian theater, even though she's not gay and the play is concerned solely with sexual relationships between black women and black men. It is not just that the play originated in a lesbian bar in Oakland, or that it was the launcher of Trazana Beverly's career. Or that Sapphire, a contemporary black icon, was Shange's student. Or that Sapphire and writer Pamela Sneed and many black lesbian and gay performers use a stance and presentational style right out of Shange's work. Or that she was published, originally by Michael Denneny, a pioneer editor of gay male publishing. Or that Shange is a beloved and welcome guest whenever she speaks at the Gay and Lesbian Community Center. It seemed to me to be more than that, which had everything to do with Lorraine Hansberry.

Hansberry was the first black person and the fifth woman to win the Drama Desk Award for her Broadway hit, *Raisin in the Sun* (the title, of course, coming from the poem "A Dream Deferred" by Langston Hughes, a black gay man). Notoriously, his estate would not let a recording of Hughes's voice be used in Issac Julien's film *Looking for Langston,* because the film acknowledged Hughes as a gay icon, resulting in a lawsuit. (Now, whenever *Looking for Langston* is shown, a significant piece of the soundtrack is blocked out, obtrusively, under court order.) Hansberry was a Paul Robeson Communist, a New School intellectual, a supporter of Cuba and SNCC, and married to a Jew. Her second play, *The Sign in Sydney*

Brustein's Window closed in 1964 on the night of her death from cancer at the age of thirty-four. Both that piece and her uncompleted *Les Blancs,* about colonialism in Africa, included male homosexual characters. In fact, *Sydney Brustein* took on black homophobia and gay sexism, failed Jewish idealism and ethnic white racism, before the gay, Black Power, or feminist movements had fully emerged.

A lesbian, Hansberry was a member of the Daughters of Bilitis. She wrote letters to *The Ladder* and *One* magazine about sexism in the gay movement and the plight of married lesbians and questioned gay "presentability" in dress as a tactic for acceptance. In a letter in her collection at the Lesbian Herstory Archives, Hansberry talks about walking down the streets of New York City and passing women who were dressed butch and wouldn't conceal their homosexuality in public. She's both ashamed of and attracted to them and wonders what the relationship of their presentation is to the question of political rights.

Aside from a tentative article by Adrienne Rich in a tribute issue of *Freedomways,* little has been stated publicly about Hansberry's homosexuality. Since the death of her ex-husband and literary executor Robert Nemiroff in 1991 (they divorced shortly before her death), anthologies of her work have begun to state as clearly as she did that she was a lesbian. Still, there has been no mention of who her lovers were or what kinds of lives they lived together. Elise Harris, a reporter for *Out,* told me that she had found one of Hansberry's lovers, an older Jewish woman who seems to have been active in the Communist movement. She told Harris that no one had come to interview Hansberry in the interim thirty-four years. And the content of her intimate friendship with James Baldwin has still not been part of public record, a record that continues to be demure even about Baldwin's homosexual life.

But it is her posthumous publication, *To Be Young, Gifted, and Black,* a collection of monologues edited by Nemiroff that brings us back to Shange and by extension to Sneed et al. For the structure and aesthetic and emotional scope of this piece set the standard for *colored girls*. It is hard to imagine one without the other. And yes, Shange's piece still manages to speak to almost everyone. But, as I watched, the New Federal Theater audience of black women, a handful of black men, three white dykes, and Don brought to a level of truth that was joyous, cathartic, and terrible, I couldn't help thinking about Lorraine Hansberry.

We returned to the New Federal the following December, and I felt that we had been wasting our time on Broadway, Theater Row, and Lincoln Center watching bad plays by mediocre white men with apathetic audiences at outrageous ticket prices. Meanwhile, all the action was down at the Henry Street Playhouse, with a new production of j. e. Franklin's 1971 piece *Black Girl*.

After twenty-four years, the play still worked. As a story of four generations of black women trying their best to *be somebody,* it jumped. It wasn't high art, like Shange's play, for Franklin's narrative structure was a more sophisticated predecessor to contemporary T V sit-coms. But it never got dull.

Surprisingly, Leslie Uggams, the glamorous nightclub singer and Broadway star, played the lead. She is one of those 1960s glitzy entertainment symbols of integration like Diahann Carroll, who never telegraphed as particularly black, especially in her professional association with Mitch Miller. But there she was, playing a wounded, sassy, fast-talking mother of three who works as a maid in a local high school and can't believe that any of her offspring can do better. Seeing Leslie Uggams swing her hips in a maid's uniform was really powerful. It spoke volumes about the realities of black women's lives with a strong subtext about what could have happened to Uggams herself if she hadn't been an exception. It also served to remind us of the kinds of roles that black women usually have to play in the theater.

By contrast, it was a formally provocative experience to attend the Adrienne Kennedy retrospective by the Signature Theater at the

Public, beginning with a double bill of two early plays, *Funnyhouse of a Negro* and *A Movie Star Has to Star in Black and White*.

Funnyhouse is a 1964 piece about a black woman writer named Sarah, who is sitting in her Upper Westside brownstone apartment being visited by various personifications of history, each of whom wants her soul. She'd prefer to pass for white, emulating Her Majesty Victoria Regina, but her dead father was dark-skinned and so she has inherited nappy hair that cannot be disguised. The play predates the Afro but has perfect clarity on the necessity for black people to love their hair. In her quest for whiteness, Sarah makes sure that all her friends are white, and she passes her time writing poems that imitate Edith Sitwell.

"I long to become even more of a pallid Negro than I am now," Sarah wails. "Like Negroes on the cover of *American Negro Magazine*."

To be a black woman stage writer in 1964 was to practically not exist. Hansberry's *Sidney Brustein* opened that same year, using social realism to address many of the same questions of identity and survival. *Sidney* had a palette of ethnic/sexual characters that did *not* include a black woman. Hansberry could not articulate herself on the stage in that context, outside of the interior life of the black family that she explored in *Raisin in the Sun*. Kennedy, like her contemporary, the Cuban lesbian experimental genius, Maria Irene Fornes, wisely went to formal invention to expose her own, unknown life. Expressing precise political understandings in formally inventive ways is a difficult task, but questions of identity are often best revealed through broken structures. Kennedy uses a repetitive technique in which every character from the Queen of England to Patrice Lumumba to a white landlady tell Sarah's story. Only when the whole world speaks Sarah's truth does her life finally start to emerge.

Funnyhouse is as much a play about the writing process as it is about race. Sarah sits at her desk, her life overrun by characters.

Even when she dies, the very white people that she invented live to gossip about her and trivialize her life. *A Movie Star,* on the other hand, is about being a viewer. This 1976 curtain raiser flips the terms of Kennedy's earlier work. For, in *Funnyhouse* black characters want to become white and emulate whiteness's most stultifying ways. But in *Movie Star,* everyone is black, even Marlon Brando and Montgomery Clift. It is a bold, transformed act of possession. It reminded me of Delmore Schwartz's short story "In Dreams Begin Responsibilities," in which a man walks into a movie theater to discover that the film is the story of his parents' life. He captures the experiences of using movies as catharsis, on which to project the content of one's own emotions. Kennedy does the same so that Shelley Winters is speaking about her father, the black nationalist missionary, while Bette Davis laments her experience of segregation back in Georgia. Hollywood is merely a reflection of the black woman artist's deep interior life.

A few months later, we saw a Kennedy premiere at the Public, *Sleep Deprivation Chamber,* cowritten with her son, Adam. The play explores the night that Adam, home on vacation from Antioch College, was arbitrarily and brutally beaten in the driveway of his own home in a comfortable Virginia suburb by a white police officer. After being violated and injured by the police, he was charged with assaulting an officer and faced a jail term. The play presents his efforts to find justice simultaneously with the responses of his mother, the esteemed playwright. Unlike the courtroom dramas depicting an accessible, fair, and coherent legal system that Americans are bombarded with on nightly T V, *Sleep Deprivation Chamber* reflects the truth of bias and injustice at the base of the legal system.

As the son (Kevin T. Carroll) struggles to maintain his dignity against a racist system, his mother (Trazana Beverly) is shocked at what her son has been subjected to. She clings to the idea that her public recognition and achievement will mitigate her son's situation in the eyes of the law. She actually expects justice to prevail.

I sat in the audience wondering how Kennedy could think that her stature would protect her family from racism, but through the author's vision I came to see how Kennedy's strategy was ultimately right and my own expectations were defeatist. After all, it takes a great denial of injustice to survive in the theater. But at the same time, writing takes constant attention to the tiniest details of living. Beverly reflected this combination brilliantly in her performance as the middle-aged artist with the eccentric intensity that comes from a lifetime of playwriting. The mother's refusal to give up, combined with her surprise at being placed in this situation, is exactly how a survivor of the theater would view the world. In the play, Kennedy writes letters repeatedly to Douglas Wilder, the African American governor of Virginia, asking for his intervention. He never responds, but she won't stop. By the time letter number seventeen is in the mail, her correspondents have become the motivational visitations of her ancestors, as their faces provide her with reminders of the legacy of courageous black people that the cowardly governor cannot join. These visions or delusions are ultimately what lets her triumph.

In addition to these important revivals, there were new plays from promising black women playwrights as well, although black women writers coming up in an era of no arts funding have consistently had limited access to mainstage productions. Don and I did get to see a production, upstairs at Playwrights Horizons, in the workshop space, of *Black Ink: Four Short Plays by Black Writers*. There were at least two remarkable things about Kia Corthron's talented and vigorous contribution, *Life by Asphyxiation*. The first occurs when Jo-Jo (Ray Aranha), a black veteran of thirty years on death row, is visited by the ghost of his murder victim, a fifteen-year-old white girl in ponytails and cut-offs (Liza Weil). It is a few days before the execution, and all she can do is berate him: "If you'd raped a black girl, no one would ever have cared." The power of the fact of that line being written by a black woman is overwhelming. It made me realize how really crucial the authenticity of point of view is. This is a line that has not been written in the many white and handful of black male scripts about death row. And if it has been, the meaning would be almost reversed. The white girl created by a black woman taunts Jo-Jo with her own aborted potential, but won't ever let him say, "I'm sorry."

The second great moment for me in this play is the relationship between Jo-Jo and his white prison guard, Andy (Stephen Mendillo). The fully realized, complex friendship the two men have built has a depth that surpasses even the earlier harrowing interactions. It makes the play, which began on fairly daunting political terms, end in surprising but convincing humanity and love between them. Jo-Jo goes to his death truly repentant, understanding exactly what he's done and what he's lost. The aging guard casually buries another of his friends. Corthron is a writer who understands complex human emotion and its political context. Interestingly, in the Hansberry mold, her play had no black women characters. But black women's experience was the voice of authority at the heart of the piece.

These plays present a universe of black women that is the opposite of the presentation in *Rent*. Crucial to the palatability of *Rent* is the message, repeated over and over again, that racism does not exist. Race is but a casting issue. There are characters who are black and who are Latin, there are chorus members who are Asian, but aside from the fact that the actors playing these roles, in every regional production, are color-coordinated, nothing in the experiences of the characters reflects their race. But, as we have seen, in works by black women playwrights, working in a variety of genres and formal choices, the experience of having lived a life as a black woman is essential to the details of their characterizations. This dramatic difference in content makes me draw the conclusion that white audiences and critics are much more comfortable seeing black faces without having to hear about the specifics of black life. *Rent*'s strategy allows a predominantly white audience to see themselves as antiracist because they are buying tickets to a show that casts black actors. Yet, they never have to hear about the consequences of race in a black person's life.

In fact, in *Rent,* race has no impact on social hierarchy. The greedy landlord, for example, is black. His oppressed, harassed good-guy tenant is a white boy from the suburbs. This switch in the paradigm masquerades as "progressive" because it defies stereotypes, but actually it obscures the real racial dynamics of New York City real estate. This creates a comfort zone for white audiences who, in our neo-con culture, are constantly wanting to assert that white people are just as disempowered as blacks. Or, even more sinisterly, that white people, like the white middle-class tenants, are more disempowered than blacks, an ideological stance that has lead to the dismantling of affirmative actions programs.

In *Rent,* a secondary black character, Benny—a gay, homeless math professor (another eccentric but artificial gesture toward reversing stereotypes)—is coded as an "activist." But his activism has no specific goal attached to it. When his lover, a Puerto Rican drag queen is dying, Benny nurses him, singing, "I'll cover you with kisses." But he never advocates for treatment or services as real life black gay men have done en masse. In *Rent,* unlike in the works cited above, his powerlessness is what makes him sympathetic to the audience. They feel sorry for him and do not ever have to face his anger or be made accountable by his actions. This depiction mirrors the mainstream press's coverage of ACT UP as loud, pointless spectacle while systematically obscuring the specificity of how ACT UP actually achieved change.

Corthron, like Shange, Franklin, Kennedy, and others is a writer whose compassion does not overcome the power of her art. Their work is explicitly the product of social and institutional forces, consciousness, highly crafted aesthetic sensibilities, and a deep look within themselves. Their plays are not Bennetton ads, where "one of you and one of you and one of you" are assembled and blandly equated to sell a product. Their antidote to Jonathan Larson's caricature adds dimension to the broad cultural expression of the racial mix that makes up American life without ever whitewashing the racially specific experiences of their characters. This whitewash is both sorely lacking in and at the core of the success of *Rent*.

TOWN HALL

Ironically, at the same moment that *Rent* was winning Tony Awards and Pulitzer Prizes, there was a vibrant discussion about theater and race going on backstage. August Wilson, the award-winning playwright, had made a blistering speech at the Theater Communications Group annual meeting in which he lambasted racism in the commercial theater. The speech was printed in *American Theater* magazine and had generated fierce debate.

On a snowy night in January 1997, Don took me to Town Hall to see the live debate between August Wilson and Robert Brustein on these issues, to be moderated by Anna Deveare Smith. Their discussion was to be about the racial separations in American theater, control of resources, and expanding the parameters of who makes up American artistic and intellectual life. The sidewalk was packed in front, people begging for tickets, papparazi hoping to catch sight of the most famous. But it was the audience that starred that night. If anyone ever thought that theater was dead, this proved the opposite. It was an audience of actors, writers, directors, critics, theater professionals, and fans of every stripe, race, and step on the hierarchy. They had all come together on a Monday night because the fact is that theater people love theater. Theater people are worried about theater. I believe that most of this audience did share a common dream that night: an artistic expression that reflects the full range of American ideas for the full range of American audiences.

This was the perfect night for stargazing. I met Paula Vogel for the first time, shook hands with John Guare, with Migdalia Cruz, saw Forest Whittaker. I was so excited I even smiled at Michael Greif, the director of *Rent*. After all, this *Rent* mess was Larson's fault, not his. I saw Henry Louis Gates, Kwame Anthony Appiah, Lani Guanier (one of the most beautiful women on earth), George Wolfe holding court. Even Arthur Schlesinger and Helen Mirren were there. The air was filled with gossip, agendas, and hope.

It was kind of raw, the way theater always is: good or bad. Real people in front of you, wanting something, showing their desire. I think that's why theater has a better reputation than it deserves. The people who make it are so vulnerable. Their desire is so palpable. Their lives are filled with struggle. Almost no one gets rich on the theater. That's why we think of it as a place for progressive ideas, as a progressive force on the culture at large, something hopeful and somewhat pure.

I began making theater in 1979 when I joined a company called More Fire! Productions, run by two fellow waitresses Robin Epstein and Dorothy Cantwell. Even though Dorothy and another company member, Stephanie Doba, are straight, our company produced plays primarily for the underground lesbian audience. We worked out of the University of The Streets, a loft on pregentrification Avenue A. We had lights made out of coffee cans, and Robin and I would leaflet outside on Saint Mark's Place, inviting anyone who looked gay to come to the show. This was a time before the commodification of homosexuality. We were part of a broad, energetic theater community with no institutional support, affiliation, or recognition.

As the years passed I continued to write and act in plays in the East Village. Except for one run of *Epstein on the Beach* at the Performing Garage in Soho, most of my plays, collaborations, and adaptations were produced over the next fifteen years in my neighborhood. The artistic ideal at that time was that you start small and grow; that you work on community-based theater and eventually you begin to win critical and financial support, get more respect and opportunity, and move up the ladder. If this was ever true, as I still suspect it was, it was no longer the case by the time we came around. The only person I know of who ever really followed that trajectory without having to do junk was Eric Bogosian. But, as the years went by we found no diminishment to the hostility facing lesbian content in theater.

So a debate about race and representation in American theater was, I extrapolated, a discussion about me. An opening up of the power structures that confine theater could only be beneficial to all of us. White male plays didn't represent me, and the general logic has always assumed that any cracking open of the power cliques has broad reverberations. I believe that, in and of itself, the opening up of white male theater to black male playwrights is a progressive step. But really I hoped that the Town Hall discussion would inspire something more.

When George Wolfe got control of the Public Theater, my colleagues and I were really hopeful. No mainstream theater in New York has ever developed lesbian playwrights with primary lesbian content, and finally here was a theater that was for the rest of us. They were a little disorganized and managed to lose scripts and take years to never actually respond. But I was still hopeful that they would be the first to define lesbians as part of the Public. It's natural, after all, to have chaos when you're reimagining the world. At one point, I did have a phone conversation with someone in Development. She very nicely and carefully explained to me that the Public was interested in diversity and wanted to show the works of people who had been traditionally excluded from theatrical production. I was thrilled. This was a great moment that I had been waiting for. This was the leap forward that told me I was right all along to insist on lesbian content, to not closet my work. The world had finally caught up.

92

"Oh, that's fantastic," I said. 'How wonderful that you want to do lesbian plays."

'Well," she said. "We're interested in lesbians of color."

I went home and I thought about that conversation. I thought about it for months. Ultimately I decided that if the Public was going to be the only mainstage theater in New York to develop lesbian full-character plays, and if that work was going to be by writers of color, great. That work would represent me more than stupid yuppie crap. So I waited and waited and waited. By the night of the Town Hall debate I had been waiting for three years, but still not a single play with openly lesbian content by an out lesbian of any racial group, had come from the Public Theater—only one-woman stand-up and solo club acts. A number of gay men, white, Asian, black, and Latin, had their work produced. Only a handful of women, all closeted or straight. White gay men seemed to have plays done all over town, side by side with the straight boys but only the Public had the broader view. My colleagues and I were the outstanding exception. Maybe something would happen at Town Hall that would mitigate all this.

Anyway, I'm afraid that like the audience, you've had too much build-up. By all reports, anecdotal and published (which rarely correspond), it was a flop. But an interesting one. The action in the bleachers was fantastic, but the show on stage was pathetic. Robert Brustein, the famed critic of the *New Republic* and director of the Harvard American Repertory Company turned out to be a hardcore dinosaur. He made clear by example his firm belief in the normalcy of whiteness, the objectivity of maleness, and the value-free nature of heterosexuality. He felt free to be as prejudiced as he wished and still retain his normalcy. Deveare Smith was just the opposite. She appears to be neutral but achieves that surface by camouflaging and repressing her experiences and opinions. Certainly, her great talents as a performer bring merit to her level of recognition, but she also achieves popularity as a social symbol offstage through this camouflaging technique. Her approach that night gave whites and men in the audience the feeling that they had seen a black woman participate in public discourse, and yet she had not actually said anything of substance. It was a relationship that can become dangerously mutually convenient.

But it was Wilson who was the biggest disappointment. While he rightfully condemned the exclusivity of white theater, he seemed to lack a freedom vision. In the end, he was only about getting straight black men into the fold. At one point someone in the audience asked, "What about women?" and he answered "I mentioned my mother, didn't I?" And he was serious! He didn't care about the dramatic lack of women playwrights or other people of color, and he absolutely didn't care about lesbian and gay voices in the theater. In fact, he said that women should not play men and men should not play women. He said this in front of Anna Deveare Smith who regularly plays men. He also said that black actors should not play parts written for whites like those in Checkov, and from our seats in the balcony it was clear that a lot of black actors booed. Basically, he lacked imagination.

But still he had my sympathy because he made his decisions rooted in personal integrity. He had used his position of authority to advocate for the underrepresented, but only of his own group. Of course, this was precisely the point on which he was vigorously attacked.

"How can you complain," person after white person whined, "when the system has been so good to you?" And Wilson never really addressed that charge to satisfaction. He let them get away with it by becoming defensive. But I think that the answer is clear. When he had no fame or power, no one cared what he had to say about the exclusion of black straight men from the American theater. He could speak all he wanted to, but no one would listen. Now that he has the power to be heard, they condemn him for not being grateful enough, for not being bought off, for not abandoning his own community. This was why I emerged from the debate with more sympathy for Wilson than the others.

When people in the audience started to yell from their seats, Deveare Smith stopped them dead. We were only allowed to ask questions by submitting them on little index cards, which she could then censor. My question was, "If this forum was about the lack of women playwrights, how many people here would have shown up?" She flipped past that and many others, and instead chose the most benign questions like "Mister Brustein, what have you learned from Mr. Wilson? Mr. Wilson, what have you learned from Mr. Brustein?" Those kinds of questions are corrupt because they assume an equitable playing field where none exists. It's like people who say, "That judge is so fair, he rules half the time for tenants and half the time for landlords," when the landlords are wrong 90 percent of the time. I guess it was the most symbolic moment of the whole affair, the talented black woman who has made it to the top of a racist, sexist art form being the enforcer of silences for the kinds of people who had no voice on that platform.

CONCLUSION

The initial reason that I wanted to discuss in depth the theatrical work presented by the kinds of people colonized in *Rent* was to make record. But the actual chronicling turned out to be a far more upsetting and indeed, *heavy* process than I'd anticipated. I'd laid out for myself the evidence that the social margins are producing the most vibrant investigative and resonant work of the culture. This makes the fact of the containment so much more painful. If we were as mediocre as they are, the whole discussion would be a different matter.

I remember in 1982 there was a demonstration of one million people in Central Park against nuclear weapons. And I have a memory, which may be fabricated, of Alice Walker making a statement that if preserving the world from nuclear annihilation meant keeping the world safe for the domination of white, straight men, maybe the world should end. This is an idea that I have grappled with ever since the day that I imagined I heard it. It represents a worldview that is both unfathomable and inexplicable to those in dominant culture because their dominance is founded upon their inability to see how it is constructed. If they had to notice how their power is maintained, their power would be diminished. One of the things I've realized while working on this section of the book is that the difference in quality between dominant-culture product and art work from the margins is substantial and dramatic. You can see full productions of funded, well-reviewed mediocre plays by white males in New York City every night of the week. Of course, there are a handful of people who question their own dominance, like Jon Baitz in his play about South Africa, but they are few and far between. Caste, not quality, is the primary factor in determining what gets produced. The current status quo for mainstream artists is stagnant and fake, involving either a complete denial of ideas from the margins or homogenizing simulacra of these ideas. The weird thing about all this, I now realize, is that they *have* to be mediocre. Only this particular falsity can justify their feeling that they are right, neutral, objective, normal, regular, as it is, as it should be, as it must be—and supreme. So mediocrity becomes a prerequisite for dominant culture's claim of objectivity, since any bit of complexity along the lines of the work I've just discussed would reveal, immediately, the injustice of their dominant position.

For this reason, in some way, Jonathan Larson needed the falsity of *Rent.* He needed to steal from a lesbian and homogenize it. He needed to falsely equate and banalize people of color, gay people, people with AIDS, and homeless people, everyone that he was not.

Any other approach would reveal a fact that he did not want to know, namely, that he had nothing to say. The possession, distortion, and conquering of people's authentic experience is the unspoken message of *Rent*. It is an assertion of the values necessary for him to maintain his delusion of Objectivity and all the goodies that come with it.

SELLING AIDS

AND OTHER CONSEQUENCES

OF THE COMMODIFICATION

OF HOMOSEXUALITY

PART 3

The particular stance of *Rent* in relation to AIDS and homosexuality is thoroughly troubling to me. At the same time, I fear that these distortions are at the core of *Rent*'s popularity.

1. Rent *claims that heterosexuals are the heroic center of the AIDS crisis.*

I have been a witness to the AIDS crisis since 1983, and I know for a fact that this is not the case. This lie raises enormous questions. How could a nation traumatized by AIDS embrace a false story about the nature of that crisis? What are the social foundations that would lead a heterosexual like Jonathan Larson to feel comfortable making these false claims and would enable the media and general public to embrace them?

2. Rent *clearly depicts a world in which heterosexual love is true love. Homosexual love exists but is inherently secondary in that it is either doomed or shallow or both.*

What is it about this moment in history that makes the dominant culture need and want an overt statement of the primacy of heterosexuality? What are the ways that this message is being conveyed while acknowledging the existence of homosexuality but diminishing it?

3. *The experiences of gay people and people with AIDS are exactly the same as the experience of those in the dominant culture.*

Why does the dominant group insist on erasing the specificities of minority experience? What is their investment in this, and how is this process being carried out in popular culture?

Key to the social anxieties and subsequent manipulations played out in *Rent* is the role of "tolerance" in contemporary American life. We, at the turn of the millenium, live in a time of great intellectual repression. This is the contradiction that filmmaker Jim Hubbard calls "freedom of speech in a country of no ideas." And many have no access to the material resources necessary to express ideas in a way in which they will be heard. The breadth of ideas permitted into the popular discourse is extremely narrow—yet these restrictions are accompanied by a rhetoric of "diversity." This contradiction, a narrow range of ideas presented as a broad range of ideas, has come to be known as "tolerance" and is now an intrinsic component of how dominant-culture people feel about themselves, how they rationalize their privileges and justify their own false sense of objectivity. Today we face a "tolerance" defined by the diminishment of the minority and the heroization of the majority, a "tolerance" that simply acknowledges that the minority exists and that claims that acknowledgement as an act of generosity. The fact that this minor recognition is the result of the suffering and insistence of millions of gay and lesbian people over centuries is completely erased.

In this section I want to explore in depth how the dominant culture is constructing a straw homosexual and a straw person with AIDS whose definition and desires recreate heterosexuals as "tolerant" without asking them to give up any of their privileges, especially their privilege not to question the construction of their dominance. For I feel that this phenomena is at the core of the creation of false ideas about homosexuality and AIDS, one small consequence of which is the production and success of the musical *Rent.*

In order to understand these phenomena, I had to look very closely at the broader content and meaning of the images and representations of gay men, lesbians, and people with AIDS that have recently emerged in the mainstream. These images pave the way for the selling of twisted history and dishonest depictions, such as those exhibited in *Rent,* to the general public. After a lot of thought and

102

conversation I concluded that the most effective and far-reaching arena for these messages was advertising, and especially niche marketing. So I begin this section with a discussion of how advertising and marketing have created a public myth about AIDS and homosexuality that is far from accurate. I hope to show how this process thereby created a social foundation that made it possible for many to accept the distortion that is *Rent*.

ADVERTISING

Advertising is our most public measure of normative standards for design, style, and the physical body. It is also the loudest, most widely heard voice on how race, gender, and age are to be negotiated. Advertising tells us what the official parameters are for beauty, sexual attraction and appeal, class, comfort, and friendship. It tells us what ownership means. It also represents the most sophisticated expression of production standards: the relationships between image and the new technologies. But, because people and institutions act on and transform each other, advertising is not a definitive mold for people's behavior and feelings. Yet it does serve as a model of normativity by which we Americans must measure ourselves. Advertising tells us to what extent each individual is a conformist or a resister, an insider or a refusenik, a native or an exile.

One symptom of advertising's dominance is that the concept of Popular Culture, as we have long been comfortable understanding it, barely exists as something separate from corporate culture. Now that marketing is so pervasive, it is hard to find independently generated codes that can escape the influence of advertising. Even slang is as likely to appear first in a magazine ad or on a television show as in people's homes. The linguistic journey seems to be reversing itself and now runs from TV writer to ad-copy writer to T-shirt producer to our most intimate discourse. It is normal for people's most private conversations about love, desire, and loyalty to include phrases and slogans gleaned from ad copy.

The targets of marketing have shifted dramatically in the last decade. Previously, we understood that advertising seized on original ideas of noncommodified people and exploited these ideas in the marketplace. For example, effeminate black gay men who gathered on the West Village piers developed an art form based on the movements of supermodels walking high fashion runways. Through the commodification process by which the stagnant center constantly pulls new ideas in from the vibrant margins, this became Madonna's hit song "Vogue." Meanwhile, the collapse of the Soviet Union inspired subway vodka ads encouraging us to "Return to the Days of the Czar." But these products were not designed to be marketed to their source audience. While I'm sure that black gay men and anti-Communist Russian immigrants did buy "Vogue" and vodka, the primary market for these products were white American middle-class consumers.

This is no longer the operative method for getting products into consumers' homes. Today, advertising relies on a philosophy of niche marketing that has become so precise that Puerto Rican girls, poor alcoholics, Christian fundamentalist rock fans, punks of Arab descent, teenagers wanting cigarettes, and terminally ill gay men all have their own interactive relationship with some area of advertising. There are fewer and fewer pockets of American culture that exist subculturally without a marketing influence. Probably the categories that remain untapped are dominated by people with little discretionary income. So, for example, even though there are now magazines that niche-market to people in prison for mail order business, there is still not a lot of advertising aimed at the homeless. Although you can imagine disposable tents and sleeping bags, body-size versions of Wash-and-Drys, and portable disposable containers for urine and feces as products of the future. While heroin,

ecstasy, L S D, and marijuana culture have all been heavily commodified through fashion, magazines, books, paraphernalia, and music,
crack culture—while commodified through music—is still not directly reflected in advertising, except through the multibillion-dollar
recovery industry. Most economically functional groups and many
borderline communities now have a direct, intimate, and deeply
personal relationship with advertising.

Take, for example, the market of people who are survivors of
sexual abuse from their parents. The social phenomenon of creating
a public discourse on the fact and impact of sexual abuse has en-
abled people who have survived it to build broad recognition of the
wrong they endured and methods for healing. And this process has
created a huge industry, not only of self-help books, memoirs, and
films but also of therapeutic techniques with the adjunct products
and services. Yet sexual abuse of children by parents has not diminished, and very few adults are actually punished for it. So in some
sense, the combination of the public phenomenon of all these incest-
related products and the continued practice of sexual abuse in some
ways normalizes incest as something that can now be discussed at
the dinner table without being eliminated. I would contend that it is
the kitsch effect, the array of accoutrements and consumer products
that become, in this case, the normalizing factor. Incest is wrong,
but now we can talk about it; incest continues unabated, but if you
are a survivor of it you can purchase all these products to mitigate
the harm done to you without society having to mitigate the practice.

The rapidity with which newly articulated identities get channeled
into marketing is an interesting one. It is a postmodern affirmative-
action employment plan—designed, not with the purpose of social
equity in mind but to give marketing companies direct-pipeline
access to information about emerging consumer niches. The campaigns are increasingly created by design teams that include at least
one representative individual from the particular consumer cate-

gory in question, who works inside the marketing industry. Their job is to take their knowledge of the source community, to engage its sensibility and wrap that around the desire for specific products, presented in such a way as to acknowledge the codes of the particular niche. The presence of these representative individuals in the industry allows for a contained upward mobility, even though the larger marketing structure is controlled by dominant-culture people. Most seductively, the presence of these individuals in the industry allows their previously overlooked or excluded community a veneer of normalcy by the fact of being represented in the marketplace, which is now a measure of American citizenship.

The classic example, of course, is the representation of African Americans on television sit-coms and in advertising. The presence of black actors provides a false image of integration and equality, especially economic equality, that is appealing to both blacks and whites. The creation of a handful of black celebrities off-screen gives the illusion that black people are participating in the ruling class, and their presence in gossip magazines, as endorsers of products, and as public figures provides a pretense of authority. But this artifice does not give any real social or economic power to black people. In a sense, inclusive advertising is less true than exclusive images were, because segregated marketing to whites at least reflected the fact of white control of the wealth of the United States. Integrated advertising is a public statement that black people now participate fully in the economy. But actually, black people (African Americans as well as African and West Indian immigrants) participate as consumers and as producers, workers, and buyers, but not as people who control the wealth of the nation. Their consumer dollars primarily go to strengthening white people's hold on their lives.

Marketing can now use the existence of nondominant experience to two lucrative ends: it can sell products directly to minority groups, and it can repackage minority expressions and ideas for voracious consumption by a dominant culture that can't come up with its own innovations. So, products that might originally be sold to a special-interest group, like leather pants to people with sexual fetishes, eventually become so palatable that any housewife can now wear her chaps to the mall. This is reflective of another shift in the function and mechanism of advertising. Previously, advertising served to repress any signs of the existence of marginal people or of a changing American demographic. Now, with new strategies of containment in place, the existence of most Americans is no longer being denied. Instead it is presented within a context that seductively normalizes the *fact* of people's lives without actually addressing any of their special needs. That different Americans might have different perspectives, needs, and experiences of American society is subsumed under one representative acknowledgment: that different kinds of Americans have different kinds of products that they can be convinced to purchase.

HOMOSEXUALITY AND ADVERTISING

We live in a society deeply conflicted about homosexuality but no longer able to deny its existence. This combination makes gay people simultaneously an ideal group for niche marketing and for the containment inherent in commodification to straight consumers.

Of course, gay men's relationship to advertising is quite different from that of lesbians. In this, as in virtually all matters, lesbians and gay men have distinctly different and dramatically divergent experiences. However, it is important to underline that while marketers are primarily focused on extracting consumer dollars from gay men, they *believe* that they are also marketing to gay women. The difference between their intent and the fact of the matter is quite instructive here, because the intent is rooted in a fixed belief that lesbians barely exist. Lesbians represent one of the few subcultures that are still too underground to be fully seen by marketers, including gay male marketers. The reasons for this are many and varied.

The Mitigation of Class by Homosexuality

Class, complex enough, is even more complicated when coupled with homosexuality. For example, gay men of almost any class can, with a specific combination of personality and opportunity, elevate their class access far beyond what they would be able to achieve as heterosexuals. Since many gay people have to leave their families and often their neighborhoods or towns in order to be gay, they often enter into a gay subculture that has more class mix than is available in their parents' lives. Interestingly, however, assimilation mediates this. The more possibility there is of being out in nonsubcultural environments like the workplace, the classroom, and so on, the more likelihood there is of class-stratified gay socializing. But, because of male privilege, gay men with economic power are more likely to be out, to socialize with and have sex with gay partners with lower incomes than do upper-class lesbians (of whom there are fewer in the first place). Gay men do give up the dependence on women's free labor that heterosexual men use as a foundation for their economic power, but they also give up having to compensate for women's lower wages. And there are significant monetary and class favors available in the homosocial economy of the gay male world.

There are gay men from poor, working-class, or middle-class backgrounds who have been able to position themselves in places of power or access because of sexual and social connections with gay men of higher economic classes. Their success far surpasses the limits of normative male heterosexual life in their classes of origin. This homosocial upward mobility is a daily part of gay life and is so common as to be virtually invisible. Just as one tiny example, I can think of a number of cases in which this process repeatedly worked in the counterculture around ACT UP. There, some working-class men were able to position themselves within the art and design worlds and for employment within AIDS bureaucracies (among others) by politicosocializing with more privileged men under the sexual rubric of AIDS activism.

For gay women, it is more complicated. On one hand, lesbian incomes are lower than even heterosexual female incomes, putting lesbian women at profound economic disadvantage. But there can be psychological advantages to economic self-determination in that the condition of one's life is a result of one's own earning power, not one's access to someone else's earning power. This feeling can elude some straight women or come to them the hard way. Female economic survival in this country can be dependent on financial association with a male's income, be it a father or a husband or boyfriend. Many heterosexual women who *live with* men *who are in the workforce* earn less money than their husbands/boyfriends do and consequently are enjoying a standard of living that is illusory, because it would not be possible on their own earning power. Many women who are involved with men who are chronically unemployed (for a myriad of reasons including, but not limited to, racism) or who divorce or abandon them must survive on a woman's income. We're all aware that women and children basically make up the vast majority of the poor in the United States. Of course, being cut off from family support contributes to lesbians' poverty, and I've heard from a number of people who have stayed in New York City homeless shelters that large numbers of lesbians are residents in them, far out of proportion to our numbers in the larger society. After all, would families be as willing to take in homeless lesbian couples as they would heterosexuals in need? But lesbians seem to have more psychological autonomy in their personal development because they are not spending their lives taking care of men and children. Furthermore, if they are of a social group in which men earn more than women, lesbians don't have to adjust to a husband's or boyfriend's employment needs in order to justify being elevated by access to his income. They often do not expect ever to have access to men's incomes and have not planned their lives around such access. Lesbians can also be more likely than straight women to refuse the poverty of motherhood on a female income, although this may be changing.

So we've already established two different categories operating in the economics of homosexuality: actual money, on one hand, which benefits people who have access to male income, and the psychology of economics, on the other hand, in which one emotionally constructs one's financial expectations and abilities based on economic self-sufficiency. In addition, given the changing U.S. economy, there is also a dramatic difference between class identity and whether or not an individual is financially stable within the parameters of that identity. In other words, one generation can be blue-collar workers in unionized industrial labor who retire as homeowners with pensions and health benefits and have blue-collar children who have none of these securities. Similarly, an immigrant family arriving in poverty could, through public education, city universities, and the GI Bill experience class mobility to such an extent that their children have graduate school degrees and work as professionals but can't save enough money to put a down payment on an apartment and have no benefits. I would argue that, regardless of class identity, whether or not a family is financially stable within the parameters of that identity has dramatic consequences on the financial position of their homosexual offspring that differ from those felt by heterosexual offspring.

For example, for gay women and men from financially stable upper-middle-class, middle-class, and blue-collar backgrounds (home ownership, pensions, retirement programs, and some insurance), homosexuality often alienates them from whatever financial support their families could or would offer to heterosexual, married, or child-bearing offspring. This can range from actual money to hand-me-down furniture to daily life expenses. For example, if your lover receives a pair of socks for Christmas from your brother, that is one less pair of socks that your household will have to pay for. If your cousin invites you and your lover to Christmas dinner, that is one Christmas dinner that you don't have to create. If your lover is excluded from the finances of family acknowledgment, at whichever level they are expressed, then you too are excluded. This condition puts gay family members in a distinctly disadvantageous financial position with respect to their heterosexual family members, that is, their class of origin. For upper-class and ruling-class families who have trust funds, significant transfers of money and property, and so on, homosexual children may be considered inappropriate recipients of family goods. Also, the family connections upon which the upper class relies may be not be available to openly gay or lesbian children or may only be offered to sons. In all examples, class background is concretely affected by homosexuality and gender.

For homosexuals whose families are financially vulnerable, within every class category, there are other manifestations of economic disenfranchisement. For example, parents who need economic help for a variety of reasons (including lack of money, old age, death of a partner) may need significant time and economic support from their children. The homosexual offspring (even if financially disenfranchised) are often the designated caretakers because they are more likely not to have children of their own. Also, they are often not considered to have a life. Their relationships, communities, and responsibilities may not read on the heterosexual scale, and may therefore result in their being expected to assume more responsibility. This situation creates a double financial burden on the gay child, most likely the lesbian, since female children are expected to give more time to elderly parents than male adult children, even though the males have more of the money demanded by such a situation. But I think that gay people capitulate to these expectations, because it is seen to be the last possible opportunity for a relationship denied by a lifetime of familial homophobia.

In many cases, it seems that in relation to society, female homosexuality is, in many cases, economically disadvantageous and male homosexuality economically advantageous, regardless of class of origin. In relation to the family, it seems that both male and female homosexuality are financially disadvantageous, with men always getting certain advantages because of sexism, which many families rely on. After all, women in the United States still earn less than three-fourths of men's income. For this reason a gay male household consisting of two men's incomes is the household model with the maximal earning capacity in the country. Even though, according to Professor Lee Badgett's study for the Institute for Gay and Lesbian Studies, reported in the *New York Times,* straight men do earn more money than gay men, gay men earn so much more than straight women as still to have a combined earning advantage over heterosexual couples. Straight men are also less likely to live together and pool their incomes. Even though lesbians have a higher level of education than straight women, lesbian women earn less than straight women who earn less than *all* men. So lesbian households have the most disadvantageous income mix possible in the United States. In other words, whoever lives with a woman loses economically. For this reason, lesbian households have the least earning power. Combine this with general emotional bias against lesbians, and the result is that we are the least likely to be targeted by market researchers.

Gay Marriage and Social Currency

It is very interesting to watch questions of consumerism and potential consumerism transform a social ideal, in this case, gay marriage.

As with heterosexuals, marriage is a very different social phenomenon for women than for men. While gay marriage may be advantageous for men, in that it will create a lawful and morally acceptable way for men to solidify their incomes, gay marriage may be disadvantageous for women. As long as women remain on the bottom of the economic pyramid, lesbian marriage normalizes and to an extent institutionalizes gay women into lives of poverty. While gay men will be able to hire women to raise their children and clean their homes, if motherhood becomes the normal expectation of lesbian life, we will be expected to become responsible for child-rearing on lesbian incomes and, as a result, lose the social flexibility that now allows us to achieve a higher educational level than hetero-sexual women. Of course, many gay people currently have children. But I am talking about the establishment of a social expectation of marriage and parenthood for homosexuals. In addition, as long as institutions of authority like courts, the workplace, the military, the health care system, education, and so on, remain sexist, the legally sanctioned but socially disadvantaged lesbian household will have a very different social experience than the gay male household. We will not be able to buy the same products and will therefore not have the same kind of citizenship.

The rendering of homosexuality into more socially acceptable privatized family units on the reproductive model, instead of the current configuration of community and non-government-imposed standards of sexual expression, opens up enormous marketing issues. While one of the primary justifications for gay marriage and parenthood is that homosexuals should have the same legal protections and options as straight people, there are also practical and emotional issues at play that translate into consumerism. If gay people had the same tax, inheritance, and benefit advantages as straight people, and — more importantly — if gay people received the approval, support, and recognition from their relatives that we long for, I believe that the demand for gay marriage would be far less compelling. Already I've observed that whenever a friend of mine has a baby boom baby (a baby, usually conceived asexually, within the context of her homosexuality), as opposed to a child produced in an earlier heterosexual relationship, the birth immediately improves her relationship with homophobic parents. Marriage and especially, Motherhood, while expensive and time-consuming, may be able to achieve what Gay Liberation never could: parental approval and interest.

While men's economic advantages are real, there is some homophobia at play in the current popular discourse about gay men's wealth. Gay men are generally assumed to have an economic advantage because they are frequently not financially responsible for children. However, many straight men who have parented children do not take responsibility for them financially. While this is widely known, this information still does not factor into the public perception of straight fatherhood. Once gay fatherhood becomes more widely recognized, the economic advantages of two men's incomes will, I predict, promote gay men in the public eye as good providers. Lesbians, on the other hand will face a different judgment, especially because motherhood tends to erase homosexuality in the popular imagination. This is because motherhood is traditionally seen as desexualizing and also normalizing, while child-rearing for men is exceptional and praiseworthy. As gay and lesbian marriage and parenthood become more normative, we may see more traditional gender power gaps between social roles for gay men versus social roles for gay women.

An added twist to all of this is the claim of Andrew Sullivan and other gay conservatives that same-sex marriage is desirable because it will promote homosexual monogamy. Again, we're being offered a traditional consumer image: two cars, home ownership, and keeping up with the Jones-Smiths' computer technology for the children. The image is comforting for heterosexuals, for whom consumerism and citizenship have become intertwined. It enables them to imagine gay people owning the same products that straight people own.

But it is predicated on a consumer whose buying patterns are determined by his or her commitment to one sexual partner each. Which is a theoretical foundation of marriage.

We're all familiar with the theoretical roots of heterosexual monogamy: from the men's point of view, patrimony, inheritance, and other practical matters; for women, heterosexual monogamy is supposed to compensate for the inequity between men and women's earning power, guaranteeing that women and children would not be cut off from the benefits of men's incomes and social currency. There also is the secondary assumption that the best possible scenario for a child is to grow up in a household with the man and woman who biologically parented it and that monogamy would keep both adults focused primarily on this structure. Of course, subsequent revelations about the prevalence of child abuse, the demoralization of female children, domestic violence, and so on, have shaken our belief in the perfection of this arrangement. Besides, we all know that many heterosexuals are hypocritical about their marriage vows.

Homosexual monogamy would be an entirely different matter. While the image of the openly polygamous homosexual does inspire distinctly different buying patterns than those of the monogamous one, homosexual monogamy is a dramatically different animal than its heterosexual counterpart. And I think it will ultimately resist the normative consumer box being promised by the gay marriage bandwagon. Partners of the same gender have more similar earning potential than heterosexual partners, mitigated of course by race and class. However, based in gender, economic protectionism is not at stake. Sullivan and others claim that homosexual monogamy will provide "stability" to homosexual relationships. But since lesbian couples, in relation to the rest of the society, are at an economic disadvantage, the most effective way to help us have stability is to eradicate the feminization of poverty.

Heidi Cowgirl, a law student I met from Corvallis, Oregon, suggests an innovative way to ensure stability for economically disadvantageous coupling. She proposes that if women, gay women and men, and people of color are going to systematically earn less money than heterosexuals and men and whites, then prices should be adjusted to compensate for the inequity. So, for example, if women earn 75 cents for every dollar a man earns, then if men pay $1.50 to take the subway, women should only have to pay $1.12. If men have to pay $1,000 a month rent, women should only pay $750.

At the same time, to imply that for gay men stability is predicated on monogamy is simply untrue. Everyone knows long-standing gay male couples who are sexually polygamous. The ingenuity of gay culture has created this possibility for gay men, one that many heterosexuals and lesbians may envy. And an equally ingenious underground economy has developed to sell polygamous sex to gay men, ranging from hustlers to sex clubs to cock rings to tours of Thailand. Frankly, gay monogamy should remain a personal decision based on an individual's emotional, sexual, and pragmatic needs. To sacrifice this in order to help straight consumers identify with a normative gay model is good marketing, because it throws in the premium of "tolerance," but also a bad argument for social change.

Gender and the Production of Advertising

In terms of the production of advertising, women in general are less likely to be in positions of power in corporations. Because of the lack of power networks, lesbians at all social levels tend to be more closeted and less visible than gay men. Lesbians, therefore, would be less likely to fill an expressly stated professional position as a niche marketer in the way that a gay man or a straight woman might. This is partially a result of being less frequently seen by the dominant group and having less economic security and fewer support structures. However, to the extent that individual lesbians identify with gay men and can read and understand the codes of gay male culture used in niche advertising, marketing to gay men can result in sales to lesbians.

Lesbians, who have spent lifetimes translating subtext and innuendo in order to have the normative pleasure experience of seeing themselves represented, can personalize advertising targeted to gay men without the advertising agencies needing awareness of their consumer profile. Interestingly, at the same time that niche marketing to lesbians is currently in this de facto state, lesbian imagery is appearing more frequently in ads for luxury items that tend to be out of range to the average lesbian consumers, who are the least likely to have discretionary income. So the marketing to actual lesbians is by default, while pseudo-lesbian images are being used to market to straights.

Of course, it is no surprise that these images generally reflect a heterosexualized version of female homosexuality instead of the authentic range of lived experience. Lesbian consumers know the language of this false imagery and easily identify it as proof that the dominant group acknowledges our existence at the same time that it doesn't know or care about what that existence consists of. For some lesbian consumers, this is reason enough to identify with a product. However, it is only gay male marketers who even consider the lesbian consumer, even if it is in a distorted way. Niche marketers to Asian women, for example, do not consider Asian lesbians to be in their consumer pool. So lesbians of color are forced to project themselves through the false scrim of a distorted white lesbian image extrapolated from a distorted white gay male image designed really only with gay male dollars in mind. This follows the pattern of Latino males, who must extrapolate from niche marketing to black males for assimilative dressing cues. For some lesbian consumers, the extrapolation connection, no matter how thin, is reason enough to identify with a product. It is seductive to see one's self translated into acceptable codes of behavior and therefore depicted in an approving way, even if the details are false and the approval illusory. It is something like the way the "You don't have to be Jewish to eat Levi's rye bread" campaign freed Jewish mothers of the early sixties from having to buy Wonderbread. Now they can eat rye bread without threatening their Americanization, because, for the first time, it came presliced in plastic and Christians were eating it, too.

As with African Americans, increased gay male visibility in advertising and adjunct lesbian sales correspond to a time of fierce political opposition to a gay and lesbian equality. Judicial and legislative oppression in many states, presidential abandonment, and the exclusion of authentic gay experience from public culture dominate the moment. Fundamentalist Christians become the mainstream of the Republican Party, right-wing militias emerge as the authentic working-class movement, preemptive anti-gay legislation becomes commonplace, and even in New York City Irish lesbians and gays are prohibited from marching in the Saint Patrick's Day Parade, as Ikea, Absolut vodka, and Godiva chocolates all vie for gay male dollars.

In 1994, in this context, I interviewed Dan Mulryan of Mulryan/ Nash, a gay-owned advertising agency that pioneered gay niche marketing. In addition to doing a lot of the basic conceptual work for this social movement, Mulryan/Nash also handled large, ambitious accounts. For example, they took on two accounts that represent a huge ideological leap in capital's relationship to gays (men). Mulryan/Nash were responsible for selling Tony Kushner's *Angels in America* to gay tourists, and they also worked for the government of Holland to develop vacation interest among gay and lesbian travelers. Both of these accounts represent new levels of recognition of niche potentials for gay men, for they acknowledge that when gay people travel, they want to consume gay culture. This goes beyond the function of the early Damron Guides or Gaia's Guides that gave gay travelers information on safe places to stay and how to obtain sex. Actually, in 1979, I worked for Gaia's Guides for four dollars an hour calling up gay bars around the country and asking if they welcomed lesbian clients. A number of places were shocked that someone in New York knew that they had a gay clientele, and a few were downright paranoid about it. But now, the recognition of full-blown gay tourism goes beyond necessity to a proactive interest on the part of gay people to see gay things.

In their 1994 prospectus to clients, Mulryan/Nash made some interesting and provocative points. The primary statement underlying their marketing strategy was the belief that "gay consumers make up affluent, educated and discerning market segment . . . [and] provide marketers with an unrivaled set of characteristics." Very importantly, the word *characteristics* corresponds exactly with the biological determinist ideas about homosexuality that were coming to the surface again at that historic moment, which predate, but helped pave the way for, the marriage trend. In order to understand the influence of the biological determinist arguments on gay niche marketing, I first want to lay out a bit about the nature of those discussions.

Biological Determinism and Economic Power

How can homosexuality have a cause? Like light and water, it just *is*. There are so many different ways to be gay that the idea of a singular source seems absurd. Most people's sexual and emotional lives can be broken down into a complex combination of biology, coincidence, and opportunity, with a little personality (a combination of all the above) thrown in for good measure. So, why this public mania to find an explanation for homosexuality? In a way, simply asking the question is contrary to gay people's best interests, because it maintains our existence as a category of deviance. After all, no one is running around trying to find out why some people like sports.

Interestingly, all the public homosexual champions of biological determinism are men. Lesbians seem to show little interest in these ideas. While the urge to explain homosexuality initially came from the heterosexual majority, gay men like Simon LeVay and Chandler Burr among others, are increasingly championing the campaign themselves. But unlike favored theories of yore, such as passive fathers, absent mothers, large clitorises, and too much/little testosterone, the explanations now favored by many gay men are genetic or neurological, while lesbians have a long history of theorizing their sexuality as a "choice," often in relation to women's social condition. After all, heterosexuality requires both heterosexual sex and heterosexual social roles, two areas with different sets of problems for different personalities. I'm sure that there are lesbian women who could function sexually with men but cannot stomach the social role. Similarly, there are women who need the social role of being a heterosexual female, but are not sexually suited to it. While some women may be in agreement with the recent spurt of biological theory, gay cheerleaders for these ideas are almost entirely men.

There are probably many factors contributing to this gender division. Perhaps Adrienne Rich was right in her classic article "Compulsory Heterosexuality and Lesbian Existence." There she argued that female and male homosexuality were dramatically different phenomena with different social consequences and different cultural meaning. Rich argued that it was homophobia that linked the two in the public mind. This division has been dramatically underlined by the emergence of the category *transgender,* which, like homosexuality, has different sociological and material conditions relative to genetic gender of origin.

Heather Findlay, the editor of *Girlfriends* magazine in San Francisco has an interesting insight into this debate. She attributes the gender split, initially, to men's confidence in science, a social force that has historically advocated for men and pathologized women. But even more influential, Findlay argues, is a long tradition in American society of attributing men's behavior to "urge," uncontrollable physical need beyond logical or ethical constraint. We're all familiar with the classic rapist's excuse that he "couldn't help himself" because of the hyperbolic power of male desire. Lesbians, of course, have given up the key to the kingdom for the sake of our twats, but we don't have a similar history of explanation. Instead, our passion has been attributed to our inherent evil, neurosis, or hysteria getting the best of our logic. "He's gotta have it" seems to be much eroticized, while "she's gotta have it" has been applied to women's disadvantage. But, notes Findlay, perhaps the lesbian version of the uncontrollable instinct is being played out in the new dyke baby boom.

Biological theories of homosexuality have been surrounded by a flurry of studies and surveys claiming to count the number of gay people in the United States. The results are treated with authority by the media, even though they are filled with contradictions. Some count a person as gay if he or she only have homosexual desire. Others require homosexual practice. Still others require *exclusively* homosexual practice. Frankly, the only thing these statistics seem to show is what percentage of gay people will come out to a person taking a survey. But the reason the biological determinists need to show a consistent percentage of the population willing to come out to statisticians is to establish homosexuality as a normal variant. Numbers that are too small imply some kind of defect, reinforcing the companion view of homosexuals as genetic mutants. As someone who has traveled through many rural and urban gay communities in this country, my anecdotal observation is that most gay people are still married. The percentage who are out of the closet and living acknowledged gay lives is very small. How do we construct surveys that measure how people would have lived without oppression? It's impossible.

Other studies are just as easily taken apart. Dean Hamer's recent claims of a gay gene are shoddily constructed. In his study group he found that more gay people had queer relatives on their mother's side of the family than on their father's side. Hamer then concluded that the gay gene was matrilineal and X-linked. However, this could be just as easily read as proof that more people come out to the women in their families than they do to the men. So mothers might be more aware than fathers of which relatives are gay or lesbian. Genetic explanations seem inappropriate.

The one great silence in all of this biological discourse has to do with *inherited* genetic traits. If we are homosexual because we carry that gene, then who did each of us inherit it from? Does that mean that every gay person had a parent who was biologically gay or lesbian, but socially coerced into heterosexuality? Most of us have a parent whom we suspect had homosexual potential. If gay-dar works on the subway, why can't it work around the dinner table? Society seems very happy with the idea that gay people are biologically apart, but they haven't realized what this says about the straight people themselves. Unless of course, you believe in acquired characteristics, in which case, maybe the experience of having integrity changes the size of one's hypothalamus.

Wouldn't society be better served by social and scientific inquiry into the cause of homophobia? If we could come to a general acceptance of homosexuality, we could do the really important work of dismantling antigay oppression. A social agreement that homophobia is pathological, that it destroys families and causes violence, would reorient the direction of all this research. Is homophobia genetic? Does biology dictate that heterosexuals just can't help themselves? In the meantime, it seems that biological determinism, like Andrew Sullivan's offer of gay monogamy, might just be the updated version of that old "pleas for tolerance." After all, what could make us more palatable to straight people than the tried and true image of men, driven by their hormones, and women, driven by their maternal instincts?

Using the Biological Model for Niche Marketing

Biological determinism has laid a lot of groundwork for niche marketing. First of all, it legitimized the questionable use of surveys as authentic grounds for assumptions about gay people. Second, it built on the comfortable dominant culture idea of gay people as *inherently* different.

When Mulryan/Nash published their list of gay *characteristics* in 1994, they focused on two crucial elements: (1) little or no competition from other national brands, and (2) large amounts of disposable income and leisure and travel time.

The most interesting element of this presentation is the fact that Mulryan and Nash, who are gay themselves, chose to represent gay men (although they thought they were representing gay men and women) as a privileged elite with more money and power than heterosexuals. While their personal experience would certainly substantiate their first claim—the lack of interest or recognition of gay men by public culture, i.e., advertising—I do not know if they actually believed the second point to be true. Clearly, they felt that presenting gays (men) as unusually wealthy, whether or not they thought it was accurate, would interest companies in engaging the services of Mulryan/Nash.

For the record, a front-page *New York Times* article in September 1994 reported that homosexual men earn about 12 percent less than heterosexual (or closeted) men and lesbians earn about 5 percent less than heterosexual (or closeted) women, who, in turn earn about 30 percent less than heterosexual men. So, contrary to the overprivileged image of them flaunted by gay marketers and the right wing alike, homosexuals are actually an economically punished sector. And of course, salary is not the only form of currency in our society. Clearly, as a result of the combination of higher salaries for straight women, straight women's access to straight men's income (by marriage), and the family and social advantages, not to mention insurance, taxes, and so on, enjoyed by straight men and women, gay people are dramatically economically disadvantaged in relation to straights. Yet Mulryan/Nash chose to emphasize the opposite: that gay (men) were ignored consumers with extra dollars to spend.

Why the interest in distorting gay men's earning power? This question just scratches the surface of the strange relationship between openly gay marketers and the dominant group. In order to achieve a business relationship in which the gay party can be openly acknowledged as homosexual, certain compromises must be reached. The two parties must come to an agreement about what specific ways homosexuals can and cannot be represented that are acceptable to heterosexuals. And the compromised images must speak to some need on the part of gay men, otherwise they will not be able to convince others of their group to hand over their dollars.

The particular compromise of the false construction of gay wealth gives something satisfying to both parties. For gay men, it awards them a badge of masculinity. They are still the breadwinners of the nation, as all good men are supposed to be. They still have male power through economic power and are thereby awarded the fruits of male supremacy that many gay men desperately want and feel that they deserve. That it is in actual dollars and cents, illusory is irrelevant. As long as everyone pretends that they have full male economic privileges, gay men can win the fear, respect, and erotic lucre of straight men's attention. This is a prize of enormous material and emotional importance to them.

For straight people, the myth of the powerful fag has historical resonance and psychological allure. Historically, dominant people have always been comfortable with the idea of oppressed people as secretly powerful. The easiest example, of course, is how for almost two thousand years, dominant groups of various stripes have convinced themselves that they were ruled over by a secret cabal of Jews. Not only does this relieve the dominant group of responsibility for the pain they have inflicted on marginalized groups, but it

124

further allows them to exercise their supremacy while falsely conceptualizing of themselves as disadvantaged. In Christian terms, this configuration requires no moral or ethical investigation, no contrition, and no redemption. It is extremely comfortable. The dominant culture's deal with white gay men is that they will be represented as though they have not suffered and as though no one has profited from their suffering. In return for this pretense, which eliminates all responsibility from heterosexuals, gay men will in turn be granted their masculinity, that is to say, their full economic power. For the lesbian consumer this offers only one option: heterosexual privilege. To the extent that a lesbian consumer can align with gay men, she can profit from the remasculinization of their image. On those terms, only, does her response to niche marketing actually appear to superficially serve certain of her psychological needs.

Mulryan/Nash's prospectus stated overtly that "gay consumers tend to be better educated and earn higher incomes than the average American." Therefore, the centerpiece of their proposal is that gay consumers are not now and can never be "average" nor can we be "Americans." They then provide a list of tables comparing gay consumers to Americans. One of the interesting elements concerning the parameters of these tables is that the choice of data used in the comparison is rooted in the most banal and normative product use. This is noteworthy in a time when renegade status or outlaw or bad-boy imagery is a staple of advertising. Millions and millions of product dollars are earned by convincing white straight young males that they are actually outlaws and therefore not responsible for the system that benefits them. The advertising offers them a way out of that responsibility without losing any of their privileges, if they purchase and display particular products that have been coded as oppositional. And many of these codes are modeled on straight black and Latino fashion and cross-racial gay style. Gay men, on the other hand, who are concretely rejected by the government and by their families, whether or not they want to be, are not described by Mulryan/Nash in outsider terminology. Instead they are defined by normative purchases. By going against the grain of gay men's real experience, both Mulryan/Nash and the corporate clients in question offer themselves and gay consumers an illusory normalcy that fits both of their needs. A similar process may explain the interest of urban black males, both gay and straight, in such Caucasian coded brand names as Timberland.

The implication of their differentiation between "gay consumers" and "average Americans" can be applied to Mulryan/Nash's breakdown of gay buying patterns.

1. The average gay household income is $62,100 as opposed to $38,450 for (what we can assume and they imply to be) "average Americans."

2. Sixty-four percent of gay people drink sparkling water as opposed to 17 percent of Americans.

3. Forty-three percent of gay people are enrolled in frequent flyer programs as opposed to 7 percent of Americans.

This mythical gay person constructed by Mulryan/Nash has the life of which Americans can only dream. They are perfect candidates for resentment. This false gay man is so clearly not living next door, not your son, not Asian, not your car mechanic, not your friend, not your lover, not you. It is a mythical, eroticized faraway Other who can never enter your world or your soul. It allows straight people a way to accept the existence of homosexuals without ever having to have their own sexual identity be implicated by it. More importantly, they can pretend away the power they actually have and falsely reposition themselves as under the thumb of rich homosexuals.

"Perhaps even more than sheer size is the prominent position gay men and lesbians hold in the fields of fashion, design, media and the arts," the prospectus continues. "They occupy a special sphere of influence and shape national consumer tastes. Gay men have been

126

credited with popularizing blow dryers, painter's pants, the gentrification of urban neighborhoods, disco music, Absolut Vodka, Levi's 501 jeans, Doc Marten's boots and Santa Fe home-style furnishings."

Notice the use of the word *lesbian* in this statement. Mulryan/Nash blithely claim that lesbians hold prominent positions of influence, but they are unable to name one significant product trend for which lesbians are responsible, such as pants for women. Terry Castle's brilliant book on Radclyffe Hall and Noel Coward discusses the cross-pollination of gay and lesbian ideas and their impact on the larger culture. But Mulryan/Nash simply added the word *lesbian* with no thought to its use, affirming again that lesbians have no reality and so anything can be stated about us without fear of refutation or calls for accountability.

In addition to the Jewish Communist-banker conspiracy theory model at play here, it is interesting to note which specific products Mulryan/Nash chose to highlight. The first item is *blow jobs,* oops, I mean *blow dryers.* Whether or not the resonance between these two terms is deliberate or unconscious, it does evoke images of poodles, hairdressers, oral sex, and flagrant effeminacy. *Painters' pants* are part of the working-class masculinity aesthetic prevalent in gay culture. *Gentrification* is the surprising entry. First of all, its appearance in the list presents gentrification as a desirable product that would endear companies to gay consumers. But more interestingly, Mulryan/Nash ascribe gentrification to gay men instead of to its real causes: the lack of low-income housing and the resulting inflated real estate market. By doing so, they give gentrification a happy, profitable result instead of acknowledging the homelessness, homogenization, and social chaos that it produces. This is particularly ironic considering that lesbians, because of their lack of economic power, are often among the primary victims of gentrification. Previously working-class neighborhoods that doubled as refuges for lesbians, such as Manhattan's East Village or Brooklyn's Park Slope and Fort Greene, become straighter and whiter as gentrification displaces low-income people. But Mulryan/Nash are using the word *gentrification* as a code for a completely different, but easily identifiable urban trend, namely the growth and development of gay neighborhoods in most U.S. cities.

Rather than seeing this undeniable trend as *gentrification,* it could also be understood as a symptom of the growing gap between gay people's sense of self and a stubborn, unchanging dominant culture. For, despite increased visibility and the illusion of improved social relations, gays and lesbians are increasingly being pushed to segregated neighborhoods in order to live with the least possible amount of threat, fear, and the resulting mandatory closeting. When we were willing to live closeted lives we could coexist more harmoniously in mixed neighborhoods. But most straight people have not been willing to accommodate our higher level of self-respect and so make openly gay people more uncomfortable for being out. In turn, we've had to choose living situations that are more geographically separate. These areas then become the basis for political progress, raising money, electing gay officials, changing school curriculums, and building openly gay businesses and social services. Because straight people have been unable to move substantially on their homophobia, gay visibility has been partially a force for segregation, perhaps as a prerequisite for certain kinds of power. But, if there were adequate low-income housing and economic development, the creation of gay neighborhoods would not inherently have displacement of the original residents as a by-product. But, by falsely naming the physical movement of gay people into urban areas where they can have a more dignified expression of their homosexuality in daily life as *gentrification,* Mulryan/Nash pretend that gay men are responsible for the lack of urban services to the poor. Even though this association is not problematic for Mulryan/Nash, it simultaneously preserves the comfort level for the dominant group while coding a political phenomenon in market terms.

Finally, Mulryan/Nash conflate two distinct trends in their list of gay popularized items. They name Levis 501 button-fly jeans, originally a working-class product, which was sexualized by gay subculture and therefore able to be normalized and commodified by the mainstream. Then they name Absolut vodka, a product that was deliberately chosen to niche-market to the gay consumer and was successfully established as an emblematic brand. So, for Mulryan/Nash, authentic subcultural seizing on a benign item and encoding it with a distinct meaning is the same as a brand name choosing to situate itself within a niche market. For Mulryan/Nash, corporate culture and popular culture are one and the same.

The ability of a product like Absolut vodka to engineer an equal level of subcultural impact as an authentic tradition emerging from the same community is only possible because of a fierce brand loyalty among gay consumers at that historic moment. As Mulryan/Nash put it, "Many gay men and women are separated from their families. . . . Therefore the mechanisms that normally lead people to choose a product are absent." For once, they are accurately assessing the lived experiences of lesbians and not only those of gay men. In other, harsher words, Mulryan/Nash notice the wholesale abandonment of lesbians and gay men by their families and propose it as a marketing device. Since our families do not want us and few national advertisers target us, Mulryan/Nash realize that ad campaigns in gay magazines give gay readers "an immense obligation to support advertisers who support them." The presence and placement of these ads do vary. But ads with explicit and direct gay content are far more likely to appear in gay magazines than in general-interest ones, although they will also appear in magazines that have distinctly homoerotic/closeted sensibilities, such as *Details, G.Q,* and so on. But they do not appear in magazines that are aimed at straight people like *Time* or *The New Yorker.* Rather than interpreting this fickleness as exploitation or opportunism, gay consumers initially saw the placement of gay-themed ads in gay magazines as financial support of those magazines. So, for example, when Virgin Airlines placed one ad in *Out* magazine, they received 250 unsolicited letters of "thanks"—the successful marketing strategy here being based on the idea that our families don't accept us but Virgin Airlines does. *Acceptance* here meaning acknowledgment that gay people exist and can be represented in advertising.

Are there any advantages to this process? Ideologically, some may argue that if corporations produce culture, positioning the gay community as a consumer group to be niche-marketed to motivates corporations to include gay images in advertising. This assures that, in the crassest American terms, we exist, although the ads would have to be on T V or in general circulation magazines for this to be effective. One of the inherent problems with this strategy, though, is that only the most palatable sector gets included, thereby distorting the reality of who gay people really are and how we really live.

Marketing, the First Priority of National Gay Magazines

In retrospect, it is not surprising that the national gay glossy magazines were so obstructive in exposing the plagiarism of *Rent,* while the local, grassroots papers were the ones to cover it. Of course, magazine people rely on their proximity to those in power in order to achieve their social currency. The result is a culture of the magazine business that has nothing to do with investigative reporting or advocacy. In this age of social facsimile, magazine culture is on the front ranks of nepotism, corruption, and false friendship, even when the magazines claim to be serving, representing, or covering the gay and lesbian community.

In general, the national glossy gay magazines feed directly into the commodification of homosexuality and the targeting of the gay consumer. In fact, it often feels as though bringing gay consumers to straight industry is the main reason that these magazines exist. As a result, there is an increasing similarity between the mainstream media and the national gay press's versions of gay life. There has been a dissolution of oppositionality. As a result, rather than learning from the community-based grassroots gay press about the realities and nuances of gay life, the mainstream straight press is now *the* model of false reporting that the glossy gay press mimics and plays up to. Since the people who edit the gay glossies today would like nothing more than power positions in the mainstream press tomorrow, they are primarily accountable to the people who have more power than they do: straight society and the closeted and straight people who run it.

At one time the grassroots gay press was run by disorganized but community-based collectives. It was chaotic, but a wide range of individual ideas were expressed. Now, the glossy gay press is a highly controlled and rigid phenomenon. Most of these magazines subscribe to uniform styles, narrow scopes of coverage, and a sparse collection of opinions. They tend to be run by an over-representation of ivy league–educated staffs, primarily accountable to their class, who are obsessed with straight people and closeted homosexuals. People who have always been openly gay and who work from a community base tend to be shunned. So, for example, a heterosexual like Woody Harrelson or a straight icon like Liza, or a gay person who got famous while she was in the closet, like k.d. lang, will often appear on the covers of gay magazines. But community-based leaders like Anne MaGuire of the Irish Lesbian and Gay Organization, or artists who have always been out of the closet like Nona Hendryx, will rarely even be mentioned. And our most important thinkers, such as Michael Bronski, have ideas that are too complex to be contained in the publications' simplistic boxes. Consequently, gay news is defined as coverage of closeted celebrities attending fundraisers while ILGO's eight-year effort to get into the Saint Patrick's Day Parade has never received an in-depth feature story. We're subjected to endless claims by famous lesbians that they are not lesbians while the marginalization of out lesbians goes undocumented. Despite the fact that gay magazines have a higher profile now and are more widely distributed than ever before in history, they represent a far narrower spread of opinion than their more grassroots predecessors. With long, ugly histories of racial and gender exclusion, these magazines easily maintain a homogenized exclusivity.

Any monthly issue can have its coverage deconstructed into who went to which ivy league school with whom, who is dating whom, which celebrity a certain journalist wants to have proximity to. Which gallery owner, which publisher, which rock star a certain journalist wants access to. Who is doing heroin with whom. This is so endemic that merit becomes almost irrelevant. Entire subjects are excluded from coverage because they are too controversial and unpalatable for mainstreaming, such as intergenerational sex, honest discussion about marriage, dependence on the Democratic Party, challenge to dominant-press misrepresentations of gay life, or any exposure of how behind-the-scenes power works. The national glossy gay press is too often simply a blue book for the most privileged and connected, with some murder cases thrown in for average readers to sink their teeth into.

Now, in an effort to win advertising from producers of prominent luxury items like designer shoes or novelty liqueurs, they have all dropped their sex ads, which are distasteful to straight companies and gay people who want to curry heterosexual favor. In need of other capital sources, they must position their readers to advertisers as people with large discretionary incomes. When you read the prospectuses from these magazines it is illuminating. *Out* claims readers with an average income of $55,000 a year (significantly less than Mulryan/Nash but equally absurd). They claim that gay men are the most "brand-loyal consumers" in the country. Simultaneously, in order to attract the upper 5 percent income bracket, these magazines simply do not cover news pertinent to lesbians, gay men of color, and older or working-class gay people. They may have token profiles of community-based leaders, but only the salaried heads of national organizations or glitteratti celebrities are the common reference points.

The waters get muddied further by the nature of these advertisers. Some of the companies who niche-market to gay people do not even have equitable health care or bereavement policies for their gay and lesbian employees. However, while national magazines like *Out* clearly exist to market designated items to gay consumers, they of course do not create how gay people feel about themselves. Just as homosexuals wearing ski masks on the David Suskind Show in the 1960s could translate into an affirming experience for the homosexual viewer because it acknowledged the existence of lesbians and gay men, these equally ridiculous images in *Out* can serve as cathartic turning points for individual evolution. But the process requires the reader to be experienced at being oppressed and have the skills for translating destructive, reductive depictions into truthful ones. Is that the best we can hope for from our national press?

In the end, the vast majority of gay and lesbian people end up with no representation of their lives in the media. Instead, we are bombarded by the A-list, white, male, buff, and wealthy stereotype that becomes the image in the American mind, of the average gay person. Even more importantly, it becomes the standard by which gay people increasingly measure themselves. This process works slightly differently for lesbian readers than for gay men because, as Esther Kaplan has observed, there is no standard preferable body type in lesbian culture. Still, the female images in glossy gay magazines are almost always extrapolated from the gay male model. So, women readers would never see female images that even referred to either their lived experiences or collective fantasy.

Ironically, Mulryan/Nash eventually made itself obsolete. According to a *New York Times* article of June 1996, national gay advocacy organizations like Parents and Friends of Lesbians and Gays are now increasingly going to ad agencies who are not openly identified as gay-owned. PFLAG went to Shepardson Stern, whose clients include Alabama Power and Times Warner. Mulryan told Stuart Elliot, the *Times*'s openly gay advertising columnist, that he was not surprised by the shift. "Madison Avenue has learned its lesson as it concentrates on niche marketing. . . . Agencies don't want to let the gay market get away." Shepardson Stern reported that their PFLAG ads are running without incident. Even the Mormon-owned TV station in Washington state is running them, which might be a good indication of how benign these messages can be.

NICHE MARKETING TO PEOPLE WITH AIDS

The current trend for new markets to be defined with increased precision intersects serenely with the separation of people with AIDS from the gay community.

Since the mainstream press has never presented truthful or complex AIDS coverage, the gay press has often been the only arena for dynamic reporting of AIDS information and experience. However, as the gay press has increasingly lost its oppositionality, magazines like *Out, The Advocate, Genre,* and so on, have now surpassed the level of falsity inherent in most general-interest publications' coverage of AIDS. Since dying homosexuals were more palatable than any other kind, AIDS mitigated homosexuality enough to allow gay men more social visibility. In part, the emergence of this acceptable consumer allowed mainstream companies to begin advertising on the pages of gay magazines. The magazines, in order to accommodate advertisers, began narrowing their parameters, determining what kinds of gay people could be represented. This meant less aggressive AIDS coverage, fewer photographs of sick people, less

134

anger toward heterosexuals, and fewer critiques of industry. The perfect foundation for the whitewashed, lifestyle depiction of A I D S in *Rent*.

While gay magazines are still used to niche-market to people with A I D S, the emergence of separate publications for people with A I D S (P W A) made that marketing easier and more direct. At the same time, the political desire to identify a community of H I V-infected people across sexual, gender, racial, and class lines also required the emergence of separate publications whose A I D S coverage would not focus exclusively on infected white gay men. As a result, the development of publications specifically for people with A I D S created enormous opportunities for niche marketing to the A I D S consumer.

"When you look at a niche group," Dan Mulryan told me, "You have to ask how that person identifies. People who identify as H I V-positive are an evolving market for consumer goods. Their spending patterns are largely influenced by their H I V status. People with H I V are not going to spend their days worrying about I R A s."

Of course, the widespread faith in protease inhibitors that has developed in the three years since the interview, despite its failure rate in 53 percent of patients with access to the drugs, fostered a whole new myth of personal finance for people with A I D S. In its continuing effort to portray the A I D S crisis as over, waning, or the fault of gay men who have "bareback sex," the *Times* ran a series of stories in 1997 about people who bounced back from their deathbeds on protease inhibitors and then set about reconstructing their financial lives for an unexpected, but now supposedly guaranteed, future. The impact of this sector's A I D S experience on consumerism has yet to be determined, beyond the knowledge that they will be spending a lot more money on medication and related products than their predecessors.

Sean Strub has lived with A I D S for more than seventeen years. He is the founder of *POZ*, a slick, glossy magazine for people with A I D S that features celebrity interviews side by side with monthly

135

updates on medicine, science, and Strub's own lab work. While *POZ* does take political positions regarding A I D S research and public policy, it does not use its pages to organize its readers into taking action on their own behalf. It is not an activist organization. Instead, it approaches activism through consumerism. By emphasizing which A I D S-related products should be supported and which companies should be pressured, it prefers to foreground the buying power of P W A S as their primary means of political influence.

This approach comes not only from Strub's background as a successful businessman and his belief in businessmen's rights to profits, it is also rooted in his deeply held emotional commitment to the idea that A I D S is not necessarily terminal, which has become reinforced by his own positive reaction to protease inhibitors. He believes that if people like himself can live with A I D S for almost two decades then A I D S is not a "death sentence." It is, instead, a lifestyle. And in America, lifestyle is normalized by the purchase of accoutrements.

It is easy to sympathize with Strub's view. The more normalized the lives of people with A I D S are, the more they are viewed as an ongoing, *normal* part of society, the easier their lives will be. The problem, of course, is similar to the homogenization of gay imagery in national glossy magazines, namely that most people with A I D S do not have a lot of discretionary income and cannot exercise the consumerism promoted by A I D S niche marketing. Indeed, the recent and hopeful pharmaceutical discoveries in treating the disease are not available to most P W A S, so how are they going to buy portable infusion pumps and the accompanying fanny packs? Simultaneously, general-interest gay magazines are also proposing a model of normalcy as a means to full social integration. The fact that many gay people neither can nor want nor should have to fit that model is a growing, yet ignored, contradiction. Similarly, recent medical advances with protease inhibitors and combination therapies are beginning to cast an artificial cast of resolution over the surface of the A I D S crisis. But, as others have repeatedly pointed out, if a glass of clean water was the cure for A I D S, most infected people in the world today would be unable to access it. As Eric Sawyer, cofounder of Housing Works, said at the International Conference on A I D S at Vancouver, "Most people with A I D S in the U.S. cannot get their aspirin paid for." The October 1996 issue of *POZ* revealed that Strub's own treatment at that time cost him and his insurance company $68,000 per year.

The advances in combination therapy created a marketing problem for a number of pharmaceutical companies who wanted to maintain their profit levels with increasingly outdated forms of therapy. For example, given the promising results of combination therapies, the official government standard of care now prohibits doctors from prescribing A Z T monotherapy, since it makes it harder for them to switch their patients to combo therapies because the patients might develop resistances. Following an uncompleted study called O76, in which doctors concluded that only 8 percent of H I V-positive pregnant women given A Z T bore H I V-infected children while 25 percent of those on placebo did the same, they have now continued to administer A Z T monotherapy to pregnant women in violation of the standard of care. Clearly, this is culturally possible because women are seen primarily as childbearers and not as people with A I D S needing services. But it also maintains a patient consumer group for A Z T monotherapy. Interestingly, the World Health Organization and other international groups are still conducting drug trials in Asia and Africa in which pregnant women are given A Z T monotherapy and a control group is given a placebo — even though the U.S. study shows that the placebo would produce 17 percent more H I V-infected children. In the United States, use of placebo in a controlled study is illegal if doctors already know which treatment is better. So, as pharmaceutical advances are increasingly consumed by U.S. people with A I D S who can afford and obtain them, global markets are quickly being developed and justified for outmoded medications.

Of course, medicine is only one part of AIDS consumerism. Lifestyle thinking promotes many more marketing opportunities. For example, in 1997 Strub published the first issue of *Mamm,* a lifestyle magazine for women with breast cancer. However, rather than evolving out of a cultural base among women with breast cancer, as in almost all representations of women within a gay male context, the presentation of *Mamm* is extrapolated directly from *POZ.* I have doubts as to the long-term success of *Mamm,* however, since women with breast cancer still do not see themselves as having a lifestyle—they see themselves as having a disease. And such a transformation may not be in women's best interest. Normalizing AIDS has many functions, including that it enables men to access more male privilege in a sexist world. Asserting the abnormality of breast cancer might be more advantageous to women, who need a change in the status quo in order to survive.

When I interviewed Strub in 1995 he had clearly been long examining the consumer potential of the AIDS market. "There is an accelerated consuming pattern when people face their own mortality," he said. "They tend to have greater liquidity—at least for some time."

POZ, consequently, has the most advertising of the current AIDS publications. With only 50 percent free subscriptions, it appears to be targeting readers with more discretionary income than the newsprint publications like *PWA Newsline* or *The Body Positive,* neither of which accept advertising and which have, respectively, a 95 percent and a 75 percent free subscription rate.

POZ, unlike most national gay magazines, does feature people of color, women, and sometimes lesbians on the cover. But the entire magazine is couched in gay male sensibility from its bright, slick design to its campy, sexualized language. Most of the contributors are white and gay, which is not true of *Body Positive* and *PWA Newsline.* Furthermore, almost all of the ads in *POZ* feature male models who appear to be young, buff, and gay, except for the ads with multiple actors, which usually include a young, buff, straight African American couple next to the gay models. The people featured in the magazine do not look sick. I asked Strub if there is an evolving marketing strategy toward people who, while they are HIV-positive, are at the same time asymptomatic and so would not identify with a magazine featuring models and subjects with physically obvious symptoms. "The fact is," Strub told me, "most people who are HIV-positive do not look sick." Mulryan concurs. "People with HIV are living longer without symptoms than ever before." Stuart Elliot supports Strub's position. "No disease-related advertising features people who look sick," he said. "Take hemorrhoid ads for example." But, clearly hemorrhoids aren't as politically and sexually charged as AIDS. The not-so-hidden message behind a great deal of AIDS advertising is that these products will make you hunky, young, and healthy, just like the normal gay people in *Out* magazine. "I have never believed that AIDS is 100 percent fatal," Strub said. "Some people are determined to make AIDS look awful and horrible, and they're angry if you try anything outside of that image."

So, just as normative advertising to the gay market provides an illusion of acceptance, normalcy, and approval for gay male consumers, normalizing advertising in the AIDS market provides illusions of health, wealth, and love to those with HIV. This is all achieved without the uncomfortable and unmarketable honest appraisal necessary for the fight against inequity. People with AIDS are no longer to be fought for, they're to be sold to.

Niche marketing to people with AIDS took its most sinister turn with the advent of the involvement of the viatical industry. These are companies that buy an individual's life insurance policy for a percentage of the return and then cash in the full amount upon the holder's death. Tax-free. As gay magazines have had to exclude sex ads that formerly funded the gay press in order to upscale and attract advertising from major corporations, they've lost the foundation of their funding. This has shifted the financial dependency of the gay press from phone sex, sex toys, pornography, masseurs, and escort service ads to viaticals.

In general the tone of viatical advertising is fairly transparent. The ads usually show young, white, well-dressed, and handsome men, either sitting alone making a troubled decision or happily playing on the beach. What these advertisements hide is the fact that most people use their settlements to pay medical bills and buy food. Both gay and straight-owned viaticals do not generally make a public show of contributing money to community-based projects, and their labor policies (domestic partnership, bereavement leave, etc.) are unknown. As of 1997, only one major gay magazine, *Genre,* under the editorship of Ron Kraft, has done an investigative piece on viatical companies.

"Everyone realizes that viatical advertising is gruesome in some ways," says Mulryan. "But they do provide a service. Whether it is completely moral is open to discussion." Mulryan believes that "whatever the market will bear is ethical."

Strub, who financed *POZ* on a viatical settlement, had a harsher tone. "Viatical returns of 20 percent are average," he said. "But many [companies] are making excessive returns of 30 percent–50 percent. Considering that life insurance proceeds are not taxable, 15 percent–20 percent should make an attractive enough lucrative business. Beyond that is usually a symbol of exploitation." However, at the time of our interview, life insurance companies were beginning to take a newly aggressive role in competition against viaticals. At that time Strub had just sold a policy to New York Life for 92 percent when the highest viatical offer he could find was 73 percent.

What Strub could not predict was the impact on viatical profits of medical advances in the treatment of A I D S. David Dunlop, "gay beat" (before they eliminated the "gay beat" in 1997) reporter for the *New York Times* reported in July 1996 that "longer life means lower return" to the viatical industry. He reported that since the Vancouver conference that year, at which combination therapies were highly touted, viatical payments had fallen by 5 to 10 percent. One company, the San Francisco–based Dignity Partners had ceased processing new applications altogether. "If treatments are effective in the long term," Dignity's press release stated, "the company's results will be adversely affected." Interestingly, the name *Dignity* is not only the title of an organization of gay Catholics who seek acceptance from the church, but is also a coded, euphemistic word like *pride* and *rainbow* that allows companies to attract gay consumers without having to use the words *gay* or *lesbian* which might turn off straight customers or scare away closeted ones. Early in 1997 Dignity's stock traded at $14.50 a share. After the Vancouver conference, it dropped to $3.28. Predictably, in the interim of hope about protease inhibitors, viatical ads have been disappearing from the pages of gay magazines and replaced by direct medication ads from the pharmaceutical companies side by side with increasing amounts of luxury item ads for designer clothes, Waterford Crystal, and expensive alcohol. However, it remains to be seen if and when the viatical ads will return, as the failure rates of the protease inhibitors become more well known.

In the meantime the viatical executives are not too subtle about diversifying. "Alzheimer's is another market that is fairly plausible," said Brian Pardo, chairman of Life Partners. (The fact that the name of his company uses references to gay marriage as a selling point might be little less sinister if Pardo wasn't a major supporter of antigay conservatives in Texas legislative races.) His is but one of the sixty viatical companies, mostly straight-owned, as of 1996 that were buying $500 million worth of policies from people with A I D S annually. So, while viaticals leave A I D S and enter into market territory created by other terminal illnesses, policy holders with A I D S may be stranded. Ironically, many people with A I D S need the income from cashing in their insurance policies in order to purchase hopefully life-sustaining treatments. Given the lack of subsidized medical treatment in the United States, the viatical company's refusal to make a purchase could, in and of itself, bring the holder to a quicker death.

So, while living longer may hurt the viatical industry, longer life for people with A I D S can mean larger profits for other kinds of A I D S-related products. For example, Strub was an early advocate of the home-testing kit for H I V status. "The home-testing kit that we are developing is going to transform the epidemic," he told me early on in the approval process. "It will double the numbers of people who know they are positive." Strub believes that there are currently more people who don't know that they are positive than those who do. Therefore the home-testing kit will significantly increase his target market audience: H I V-positive asymptomatics who are ready to liquefy their assets. The message that new protease inhibitors are most effective with early diagnosis further stimulates the home-testing market. This adds another category of A I D S consumer to the roster. We already have shown that people with symptomatic H I V/A I D S and those with asymptomatic H I V/A I D S have different buying patterns that have been identified by marketers. But we can now add people who *think they might be positive* as new consumers in the A I D S marketplace. These people will purchase home-testing kits, perhaps more than once. If they are positive, they will move over into the asymptomatic consumer category. The earlier people become aware that they are positive, the sooner and longer they will be encouraged into asymptomatic spending and buying patterns.

The kits were finally approved in May 1996 and by July, Johnson & Johnson, a major American corporation, was involved in a protracted court fight over the ownership and distribution rights. They were originally developed in the 1980s and sold to Johnson & Johnson in 1993. The inventor, Elliot Millenson, is a major donor to Newt Gingrich, the antigay Republican leader of the House of Representatives. The kits are called Confide, a name that is harmonious with traditional names of discreet gay bars like Secrets, Whispers, and so on. However, Confide failed to generate the kinds of sales that Johnson & Johnson anticipated, and, in the summer of 1997, the company was threatening to pull the product from the market.

In some ways, the most painful and complex element of niche marketing to people with AIDS is the role of gay people, ourselves, in making possible such overt profiteering off our own experiences of illness, abandonment by our families, and justified insecurities about our place in American society. After all, the illusion of normalcy without the fact of normalcy is the centerpiece of niche marketing to people with AIDS. It is very seductive for gay people to confuse the presence of limited gay images in advertising with some kind of social equity, but it is entirely illusory. There is no corollary between appearing in advertising and social or political power. We want our recognition by marketers (gay and straight) to be synonymous with a broad social recognition of our realities but, in truth, it has the opposite effect. Just as there is no corollary between the cultural cache of *Rent* and real political power for people of color, gay people, and people with AIDS, cynical niche marketing to people with AIDS is currently disconnected from the broad needs of people with AIDS. These gaps in credibility, while destructive, are by now commonplace and a painful manifestation of how truly vulnerable gay people and people with AIDS really are.

CONCLUSION: THE CREATION

OF A FAKE, PUBLIC HOMOSEXUALITY

This is my ninth book, and I feel that it is the most radical thing I have ever written. Yet it was made in the most conservative time in which I have ever lived. As a result, I have never in my life been so afraid to say what I know to be true.

This fear is grounded somewhat in the fearfulness I've observed during the whole process of seeking redress for the plagiarism of my novel. I've seen a lot of people back away from saying or acting on what they knew to be true because they were afraid of or identified with the corporate power of the people behind *Rent*. But that kind of thing has usually not ultimately affected me. I remember the wise words of my mentor Maxine Wolfe when she told me that radicals must never stop ourselves because we fear that a greater power would punish us. We must go forward with what we believe to be true and make *them* stop us.

But this time, my fear is located in the knowledge that the central theme of this book is systematically obstructed and denied in our society in this historic moment. Namely, that the dominant culture's power relies on their inability to see how it is constructed, that they rely on *feeling* that their power is a naturally objective state, and that efforts to articulate and analyze how their dominance is enforced are met with annihilation. This method by which our ideas are crushed takes many forms, including ridicule, exclusion, disregard, neglect, scorn, sabotage, poverty, obscurity, marginality.

Therefore, if you are naturally a political person, as I am, envisioning the concrete process of change and articulating that in your artwork is unavoidable. It is organic. Those of us who actually want a better future must take time to think about what it would look like and how to get there. Otherwise we won't get there. This practice doesn't make up the totality of our creative work but neither does it diminish it. In America, politically thoughtful artists are looked down on. "That's not art." Most published fiction in this country is passively supportive of the state. It is the kind of artist/government relationship that Americans only condemn when it happened in places like East Germany. For us, art that exposes uncomfortable truths is diminished for being *didactic,* while art that presents a false veneer of comfort is considered neutral and is promoted. Nowhere is this division more evident than in the commodification of art about A I D S.

We are in a very tender moment when society is making a transition in its understanding of A I D S from lived experience to packaged image, when *Rent* is selected over Diamanda Galás's *Plague Mass,* Derek Jarman's *Blue* — indeed, when *Rent* is selected over a novel with the same characters, events, and dynamics that does not lie about the power differentials between heterosexuals and homosexuals. As we have shown, the existence of homosexuality is no longer being denied. Instead, a fake public homosexuality has been constructed to facilitate a double marketing strategy: selling products to gay consumers that address their emotional need to be accepted while selling a palatable image of homosexuality to heterosexual consumers that meets their need to have their dominance obscured. Rather than elevating the centuries-old underground gay and lesbian culture to the level of mainstream visibility, straight people have invented their own homosexual culture and placed it front and center. As of this writing, Winter, 1998, the components of this fake public homosexuality are rigid.

146

1. Gay and lesbian celebrities are allowed to emerge as long as they become famous while they are in the closet and then come out.

2. Gay content is permissible if it focuses on romance.

3. Mild homoeroticism in heterosexual paradigms is permissible. Preference is given to "gender-bending," where one or more heterosexual party thinks they have a gay attraction but their *objet d'amour* ends up being straight, but in drag.

3. Homophobia is unmentionable. Nothing that would express anger at straight people or illuminate the pain that straight people have caused, or that would show straight people's complicity or responsibility in relation to homophobia is permitted.

4. Gay people are rarely allowed to be the heroes unless they are tragic heros, rescued by straight people. Straight audiences must not be expected to universalize to a gay or lesbian protagonist unless they have already built a relationship with that character, thinking they were straight. The most appropriate role for gay or lesbian characters is as sidekicks.

Gay-produced artwork that violates these rules is pushed to the margins. Gay-produced artwork that conforms to these rules can now be elevated to the slightly risqué environs of mainstream culture. The best and most important gay artwork, we're being told repeatedly, is made by straight people and strictly conforms to these restrictions.

The authentic work that gay and lesbian artists have done on AIDS has been replaced in the public discourse by a clean version of crisis. Vehicles like *Rent, Philadelphia,* and other AIDS stories promoted by straight people portray a world in which heterosexuals have nothing to account for, to reflect on, or to regret in their behavior toward people with AIDS and gays and lesbians in general. The role of government and pharmaceutical companies is mythologized within the expectations of the general public, and AIDS is comfortable, cathartic, or over.

Rent, of course, is the focus of this inquiry, and it might be helpful to look at *Rent* in terms of the marketing issues discussed thus far. *Rent* functions along the most sophisticated lines of the construction of a fake public homosexuality in a way that works with both gay and straight audiences.

At the center of *Rent* are two white straight men who are roommates. Ordinarily, an AIDS drama would feature two gay white men who live together as lovers, but this unexpected yet important switch immediately puts the audience at ease. It is a paradigm they recognize from other AIDS dramas. For straight audiences, who have worn out their ability to feel sorry but not responsible for gay men with AIDS, the recognition of straight protagonists is a huge relief.

The audience quickly learns that one of the straight white men has AIDS and has a straight Puerto Rican girlfriend who also has AIDS. This is also a point of relief to the white, well-to-do theater-going New York audience. After all, they think of themselves as sophisticated, not prejudiced, and here they have a nice Hispanic girl in the lead role. Oh, she's playing a junkie? Good. That's believable.

Oh, here comes the stretch. There are subplots. One involves a nice-looking black man and his Puerto Rican, homeless, HIV-infected transvestite lover. They kiss on stage while the transvestite is wearing a dress. The audience is reconfirmed in their own sense of how tolerant they are. Gay men wear dresses. They die. How sad. What a relief. Well, that's what happens to gay people, I guess. They're secondary subplots. That's their place, even in the story of AIDS.

The hero, the single white straight man, does not have AIDS. To make him even more sympathetic, he has lost his girlfriend to a black woman. He embodies the gentle straight white man whose sexual relationships and support structures are threatened by the encroachment of uppity people of color and the threat of homosexuality. He is the personification of the Theater of Resentment.

148

Nonetheless, he still gets to prove his boyish masculinity. The black lesbian is from a rich diplomat's family, and she owns a lot of audio equipment, but she doesn't know how to use any of it. Fortunately, the straight white boy who doesn't have AIDS shows her how. Her girlfriend, Maureen (his old girlfriend), should have stayed with him because she and her lover fight all the time. Bicker, bicker, bicker. They never have fun or help each other or transform each other in the way that the heterosexuals do when they're in love. Furthermore, Maureen keeps flirting with her ex-boyfriend in front of her new girlfriend, so how committed to homosexuality can she really be? Once again the audience is confirmed in their own liberalism. They watched a lesbian couple in a play! Lesbians don't have real love and don't have loyalty and can't fix their own audio equipment. What a relief.

In the end, the audience is reinforced in their own sense of how progressive they are, they are the epitome of tolerance. After all, they watched black people, homeless people, drag queens, and lesbians. In fact, they've been watching characters just like these characters on TV sitcoms, in movies like *Philadelphia,* and in ads for Ikea. And in the end, the presence of all these exotic others proved one hugely important thing, more important even than how tolerant the audience is. In the end, *Rent proves* the supremacy of the white straight people. The people who know how to love. The people who know how to live.

And what about the gay audiences? The audiences who were niche-marketed to through puff piece features in *The Advocate* and *Out*? This part of the picture is one that can be clearly understood if you really know the nuances of what gay people have experienced over the last twenty years. I say this because the gay audience at stake is principally my generation. We are a confused group of queers. In many ways we are the ones who have experienced the most dramatic and traumatic shift in public depiction of homosexuality. We had such profound oppression experiences in childhood that they can qualify as trauma. We are the last of the dirty-dark-secret generation. We are the last group that came of age in a time in which homosexuality was never mentioned, had no public representation. We were all alone as teenagers; our families punished us severely for our homosexuality. We grew up into an already existing, but fairly underground gay movement. And now we're being told to buy rainbow tumblers. It's something like my grandmother who had to share one pair of shoes in Russia and later watched color T V in New Jersey. You might say it's trading one kind of hell for another, but that's the human condition. My point is that we have experienced changes that are too huge to digest and often too confusing to fully comprehend. So, when we walk into a theater and see two women kissing on stage after we've been humiliated and vilified by our own families for doing the same thing, we're thrilled. But, in the context of contemporary culture, where Roseanne kissed Mariel Hemingway on prime-time T V, that kiss does not have the meaning that we once dreamed it would. It does not mean that we are full human beings whose lives can now be truthfully represented among the selection of lives that make up the American experience. What it really means is that, while in the past we could not be represented because the fact of our existence would mitigate the supremacy of heterosexuality, marketing and the commodification of our experiences has now made it safe for us to be represented and have that fact reinforce the superiority of heterosexuality. Because marketing has changed the codes around homosexuality so dramatically, gay people, even in their thirties, can have perceptions that are out of date with the actual meanings of certain images in today's culture—images that were once loaded but are now benign. They may not be benign to the gay person who longed for those images in the past, but in today's marketplace they mean almost nothing. In other words, marketing has done its job, diminishing the impact of a simple representation of homosexuality, and putting it to work for the heterosexual majority.

150

It's a state of mind somewhere between post–traumatic stress syndrome and what film theorist Patricia White calls "retrospectatorship," which she describes as "the recognition of the subjective implications of our past . . . our history or biography . . . that determines our current affective experiences." Emotionally, we're living in the past where we each had a profoundly unjust and unresolvable oppression experience, but we're shopping today.

What is clear is that there are two concurrent marketing trends going on at the same time. While fake stories about AIDS that make straight people feel good are the most public narrative, reaping huge financial rewards, Oscars, Pulitzers, and whatnot, real gay people and real people with real AIDS are on an entirely different consumer pipeline, invisible to straight people, where they are subdivided into more and more precise niches while losing and being denied public services and advocates. Their potential advocates, the straight people who make up their families, coworkers, and neighbors, are off to the movies and the theater. There, they are being told over and over again that they have behaved excellently during the AIDS crisis. That in fact, they are the heroes of the AIDS crisis. That gay and lesbian people are not only secondary to them but enormously grateful to them and that they have nothing to account for or even think about or notice.

This is the environment in which we are currently attempting to articulate the actual lived experience of homosexuality and AIDS. The marketplace is filled with pumped-up distortions, while the real truths are always in flux and hard to depict.

This is one of the historical trends that converged on the moment that created the megahit, *Rent*.

INDEX

154

155

156

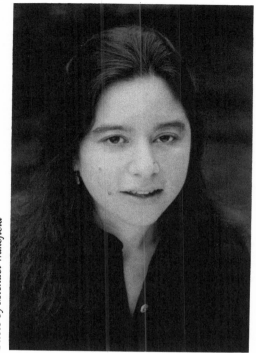

Sarah Schulman is an award-winning playwright, novelist, and nonfiction writer. She is the author of seven novels, including *After Delores, People in Trouble, Rat Bohemia,* and, most recently, *Shimmer,* and the nonfiction work *My American History: Lesbian and Gay Life during the Reagan/Bush Years.* A longtime activist, Schulman was one of the first members of ACT UP in New York and a cofounder of the Lesbian Avengers. Over the past twenty years she has contributed to numerous publications, including the *Village Voice,* the *Nation,* the *New York Times, Gay Community News,* and *Interview.* A recipient of the 1997 Stonewall Award, Schulman lives in New York City.

Library of Congress Cataloging-in-Publication Data

Schulman, Sarah.
Stagestruck : theater, AIDS, and the marketing of gay America /
Sarah Schulman.
p.   cm.
Includes index.
ISBN 0-8223-2132-7 (cloth : alk. paper). —
ISBN 0-8223-2264-1 (paper : alk. paper)
1. Larson, Jonathan. Rent.   2. Musicals—United States—History and
criticism.   3. Homosexuality and literature—United States—History—
20th century.   4. Politics and literature—United States—
History—20th century.   5. AIDS (Disease) in literature.   I. Title.
ML410.L2857S38   1998
782.1′4—dc21   98-12053